Teaching Health Professionals Online

Teaching Health Professionals Online

FRAMEWORKS AND STRATEGIES

Sherri Melrose, Caroline Park,
and Beth Perry

AU PRESS

Published by AU Press, Athabasca University
1200, 10011 – 109 Street, Edmonton, AB T5J 3S8

ISBN 978-1-927356-65-4 (print)   978-1-927356-66-1 (PDF)   978-1-927356-67-8 (epub)

Cover and interior design by Sergiy Kozakov.
Printed and bound in Canada by Marquis Book Printers.

Library and Archives Canada Cataloguing in Publication

Teaching health professionals online : frameworks and strategies /
Sherri Melrose, PhD, Caroline Park, PhD, and Beth Perry, PhD.

Includes bibliographical references and index.
Issued in print and electronic formats.
ISBN 978-1-927356-65-4

1. Medicine—Study and teaching. 2. Medical education—Computer-
assisted instruction. 3. Medicine—Computer-assisted instruction. 4.
Web-based instruction. 5. Internet in education. 6. Distance education. I.
Melrose, Sherri, 1957-, author, editor of compilation II. Park, Caroline L.
(Caroline Louise), 1948-, author, editor of compilation III. Perry, Beth,
1957-, author, editor of compilation

R834.T42 2013   610.71   C2013-905415-4
                                       C2013-905416-2

We acknowledge the financial support of the Government of Canada through
the Canada Book Fund (CBF) for our publishing activities.

   Canadian   Patrimoine
                        Heritage   canadien

Assistance provided by the Government of Alberta, Alberta Multimedia
Development Fund.

Government

To our students, who teach us to be better teachers and better people

To our colleagues, who inspire us with their dedication to teaching excellence

To our university, for giving us the freedom to be innovators

To our families, for providing us with encouragement and purpose

CONTENTS

ACKNOWLEDGEMENTS

The inspiration for this book came first from our students, who challenge us to become better teachers and often serve as a test population for new teaching strategies. Their criticisms and suggestions have helped us refine many of the ideas presented here.

We are also grateful to our colleagues in the Faculty of Health Disciplines at Athabasca University—inspiring educators who continually refine their teaching approaches. Many of them responded generously to our call for information about teaching techniques and activities that they have found to be productive and that we might include in this book. We extend our sincere thanks to Carol Anderson, Diana Campbell, Cheryl Crocker, Sharon Moore, and Joyce Springate for their contributions. Finally, a special thanks to Katherine Janzen, with whom the theory of quantum learning originated and who graciously agreed to write a chapter for the book on that topic.

Introduction

You are a teacher at heart. Your goal is to inspire students to excel professionally in one of the many health disciplines. Your students may be nurses, social workers, dietitians, physiotherapists, occupational therapists, chiropractors, dental hygienists, or radiation therapists, or they may be learners who have not yet entered their chosen health care profession. You teach at least some of your courses online, and you find it challenging to be effective, personally engaging, and "real" to students when teaching via the Internet. If this is your story, this book is for you.

Our aim is to equip health care educators, whether they are new to teaching online or already have some experience in that area, with a variety of effective (and proven) online teaching strategies and learning activities. The book offers teaching techniques that can be put into practice immediately and generally demand little by way of technological skill, the investment of time, or other resources. Teachers who find themselves at a loss for inventive ways to challenge their students can flip through these pages, scan the activities, and find an idea to suit their purpose.

This book is both practical and theoretical. It is often helpful to understand why certain teaching strategies are effective in engaging learners. The teaching activities and techniques included in this book are therefore presented in the context of contemporary educational theory, supported by scholarly literature. Teachers often struggle to understand how theories such as constructivism or connectivism or transformative learning apply to actual learning situations. By linking specific theories to concrete examples of teaching activities, this book aims to demystify theory. It is our hope that after reading this book, instructors will be comfortable discussing educational theory and may even be inspired to develop their own teaching activities based on educational theories that align with their personal teaching philosophy. Educational theory kindles ideas and inspires us to improve our teaching.

The teaching strategies and learning activities presented in this volume are drawn from the practice of many professors, instructors, and tutors who currently teach online in the Faculty of Health Disciplines at Athabasca University. Athabasca University was Canada's first open university, and, today, most of its courses are taught online. The Faculty of Health Disciplines boasts about 2,000 undergraduate and 1,500 graduate students, as well as some forty professors, instructors, and tutors who have a combined total of many years of experience with online teaching. (Many of the courses offered in the Faculty of Health Disciplines have been taught online for a decade or more.) When we set out to write this book, we solicited input from colleagues in the Faculty of Health Disciplines, asking them to share their most successful online teaching strategies and activities. We also included techniques that we have developed and found effective in our own teaching. Once we had an assemblage of activities, we grouped them according to the educational theory with which they were most closely aligned. Of course, in developing teaching techniques, instructors often integrate elements drawn from a variety of theories. For the purposes of this book, however, we assessed the "best fit" in order to illustrate the relationship between practice and theory. This book is very much a collaborative effort. However, we chose to divide up the primary responsibility for specific chapters according to our individual areas of interest and theoretical expertise. Thus, chapter 1, on instructional immediacy, is principally the work of Sherri Melrose. As she explains, the theory of instructional immediacy holds that demonstrating availability, projecting warmth and friendliness, and taking time to get to know students as individuals all play a major part in an instructor's effectiveness. Her discussion of the theory is followed by suggested ways in which teachers can encourage collaboration while also supporting individual learners as they progress through the expected stages of development in class groups.

Invitational theory is the focus of chapter 2. In it, Beth Berry discusses "the plus factor," a way of thinking and being with students that creates a warm and welcoming online educational environment. She examines how trust, respect, optimism, and intentionality exert a positive influence on educational outcomes.

In chapter 3, Sherri Melrose reviews constructivist thinking, a teaching approach that builds on what learners already know. She describes ways in which teachers can provide learners with the scaffolding, or support, that they need in order to progress toward competence and independence.

The theory of connectivism stresses the role of networks in learning. As Caroline Park explains in chapter 4, in a connectivist approach, teachers and students use digital technology to create complex and diverse networks of people who can help them find the information they need. She offers connectivist techniques that can help learners to create informal and perhaps unexpected connections that support their specific learning needs and interests. In addition to locating information, however, students must learn to organize the information they gather and evaluate it critically.

In chapter 5, Park turns to the concept of transformational learning, which she describes as a process of changing learners' attitudes and deeply entrenched beliefs and assumptions. When teachers provide learners with opportunities for critical reflection and challenge them to question commonly accepted truths, exciting new perspectives can be gained.

Chapter 6, contributed by Katherine Janzen, concerns the theory of quantum learning. Janzen draws from principles of quantum physics to illustrate how the basic elements of virtual classrooms—teachers, students, and course content—are connected and entangled, just as electrons are. She explains how teachers in quantum learning environments can create virtual classrooms that feel real and alive.

In the concluding chapter, we describe the six principal lessons we have learned about how to make online courses more engaging. Fundamentally, we acknowledge that wonderful online teaching strategies alone do not inevitably lead to success. The teacher matters. Online teachers, however, face special challenges. How can online teachers ensure success? How can they transcend the emptiness of cyberspace to become real to students and create learning environments in which classmates become as tangible to one another as they would be if they were sitting side by side? This final chapter addresses these questions and provides online teachers with important takeaway messages.

We acknowledge that online education changes at a breathtaking pace. With each new technology, fresh teaching approaches become possible. To be on the cutting edge in the dynamic world of online education, we focus here on the most contemporary of learning theories, theories that are likely to remain relevant as Web 3.0 technologies continue to emerge. The importance of social media in online education is also given consideration throughout the book. Some of the teaching strategies described use social media as the primary platform for learning, and many of the suggested activities can be adapted to employ social media as needed.

Future online learning will undoubtedly be more open, mobile, and flexible than it is today. Open educational resources, the adoption of mobile devices, free online tools and courses, and the rise of cloud computing are four trends that will propel changes in online teaching and learning. This book provides a foundation that will enable you to make optimal use of these and other transformations that will shape online learning in the years ahead.

If you are a novice online teacher, this book is a place to start. If you are a seasoned educator who has just been asked to convert some of your face-to-face courses to online courses, read this book first. If you have been teaching online for years and feel that you are "rusting out" and getting stuck in your old ways, our theory-based techniques and activities may refresh your teaching. If you are a highly regarded online teacher emulated by others, we hope that you will find some hidden gems in this book that will help you to continue to be a leader in online education.

In sum, the purpose of this book is to inspire great teaching by providing you with theory-informed techniques and activities to help make you an exemplary online educator. The end result will be enhanced quality of education, increased student success and satisfaction, and, ultimately, the best possible health care professionals.

I

Instructional Immediacy: The Heart of Collaborating and Learning in Groups

Exemplary teachers generally have one thing in common: their classes bustle with activity as students connect and interact with one another. As teachers who love what we do, we want students to share our excitement and to become fully engaged members of our class community. We know how connections among students can sustain motivation and deepen understanding of course material. But we also know how full life can be for students and how stretched their time is as they juggle family, work, and study commitments. Looking through the eyes of adult learners, we can see that carving out time to collaborate with classmates in an online course may not stand out as a priority. How, then, can we begin to foster the kind of collaboration that our students need in order to fully engage in online courses?

Albert Mehrabian's explanation of the construct of immediacy, together with theories of how groups work, offers important directions. This chapter explains instructional immediacy, provides a primer on how groups work, and suggests ways to invite students to collaborate in groups by modelling their achievements. Instructional immediacy is at the heart of collaborating and learning in groups. Teachers must demonstrate what intentional commitment to collaboration actually looks like before they can expect students to interact in meaningful ways with their classmates.

BACKGROUND THEORY

An Explanation of Instructional Immediacy

Understanding the construct of instructional immediacy is foundational to effectively fostering collaboration among students. Encouraging learners to engage in collaborative activities with one another begins with communicating our own availability, friendliness, and willingness to connect in personal ways with our students. As technology offers increasing possibilities for electronic communication, teachers must not lose sight of the basic feelings and responses that we know exist within the teacher-student relationship. Teachers who demonstrate immediacy in their classrooms, whether face to face or online, engage students and invite them to risk looking at the world in new ways.

The construct of immediacy was introduced in the 1960s by social psychologist Albert Mehrabian, who defined immediacy as an affective expression of emotional attachment, feelings of liking and being close to another person (Mehrabian, 1967, 1971; Wiener & Mehrabian, 1968). Immediacy, in other words, is a sense of psychological closeness.

In the context of face-to-face university classrooms, the definition of instructional immediacy was further developed to include nonverbal manifestations of high affect such as maintaining eye contact, leaning closer, touching, smiling, maintaining a relaxed body posture, and attending to voice inflection (Andersen, 1979). Verbal expressions of immediacy include using personal examples, engaging in humour, asking questions, initiating conversations, addressing students by name, praising students' work, and encouraging students to express their opinions (Gorham, 1988). Links among teacher immediacy, student motivation, and affective learning have consistently been documented (Baker, 2010; Christophel, 1990; Christophel & Gorham, 1995; Gitin, Niemi, & Levin, 2012; Witt, Wheeless, & Allen, 2004).

However, in electronic learning spaces, where nonverbal cues may be less clear or even nonexistent, establishing instructional immediacy, or psychological closeness, can be challenging, but it is not impossible: research has demonstrated links in online learning environments between instructors' immediacy behaviours, on the one hand, and student satisfaction and instructional effectiveness, on the other (Arbaugh, 2001; Hutchins, 2003; Walkem, in press; Woods & Baker, 2004). The experience of liking and feeling close to instructors can lead to positive effects in online classrooms (Hess & Smythe, 2001), and correlations between immediacy and affective learning have been identified (Baker, 2004; Russo & Benson, 2005).

In essence, instructional immediacy online refers to the extent to which teachers are able to project an affect of warmth and likeability in their communication with students (Melrose, 2009). In online learning environments, one-way immediacy can be demonstrated through word choice. For example, online teachers who refer in their messaging to "our" class and indicate a willingness to work "with" learners through their word choices signal qualities that may prompt immediacy. Words that communicate a genuine interest in getting to know each class member as a unique individual can create a feeling of safety. This equips instructors with the foundation needed to encourage learners to extend that teacher-student immediacy toward collaboration in the class group.

Research with online health care graduate students that explored their perceptions of instructional immediacy showed that learners value instructional behaviours that model engaging and personal ways of connecting, that maintain collegial relationships, and that honour individual learning accomplishments (Melrose & Bergeron, 2006). Examples include instructors posting self-introductions that include pictures and appropriate personal and professional information, creating a course document incorporating biographical information for each member of the class, and choosing words with gentle connotations (Melrose & Bergeron, 2006). By projecting an affect of warmth and immediacy in our own communication, we can begin the process of creating an engaged and appealing online learning environment where learners feel recognized as individuals and experience a sense of belonging to a vibrant class group.

A Primer on Groups and How They Work

In addition to intentionally projecting an affect high in warmth to strengthen individual relationships with learners, instructional behaviours that communicate immediacy also set the stage for nurturing student-to-student relationships within the learning community. Here, an appreciation of how well-functioning groups work is important. Individuals who join together in a group for a specific purpose such as engaging in a learning activity can be expected to progress through predictable stages. Social psychologists Bruce Tuckman, David Johnson, and Frank Johnson provided seminal frameworks. Tuckman (1965) and Tuckman and Jensen (1977) assert that functional groups move through five stages: forming (characterized by anxiety and uncertainty about belonging), storming (characterized

by competition, individuality, and conflict), norming (characterized by attempts to resolve earlier conflicts and clear expectations of
behaviours and roles), performing (characterized by cooperation and
productive work), and adjourning (characterized by termination and
disengagement from the group). Johnson and Johnson (1997, 2009)
identify seven stages through which functional groups progress:
defining and structuring procedures and becoming oriented, con-
forming to procedures and getting acquainted, recognizing mutual-
ity and building trust, rebelling and differentiating, committing to
and taking ownership of the goals of other members, functioning
maturely and productively, and, finally, terminating.

In online classroom environments, functioning groups are
expected to progress through similar stages (Jaques & Salmon, 2007).
Gilly Salmon (2000) identifies five stages of online group development: access and motivation (characterized by welcoming and
encouraging), online socialization (characterized by familiarizing
and providing bridges between cultural, social, and learning environments), information exchange (characterized by facilitating tasks and
supporting use of learning materials), knowledge construction (characterized by facilitating process), and development (characterized by
supporting and responding). In addition, Salmon emphasizes that the
ability to guide online groups is more important than making pol-
ished instructional presentations.

Melrose and Bergeron (2007) link the three overarching stages
of group development, beginning/engagement, middle/encourage-
ment, and ending/closure, and suggest specific online instructional
approaches to facilitate progress at each stage. For example, in the
beginning/engagement stage, learners value knowing that their
instructors are available "if you need me" and that it is "safe" to contact them. In the middle/encouragement stage, learners appreciate
personal help with networking and with managing conflict, particularly in relation to participation and marking. In this middle stage,
students also value individual private feedback from instructors. And,

in the ending/closing stage, learners need opportunities to debrief and reflect.

Implementing teaching actions at the most opportune time, such as intervening promptly when the expected conflict emerges once a group has entered its working phase, offers important reassurance to students. In contrast, implementing a teaching action at an inopportune time can have the opposite effect. For example, during the beginning phase of group work, introducing activities that encourage overlong reflection (which leads to inaction) can inadvertently communicate teacher abandonment. Knowing that learners value debriefing time in the ending stage of their group work leads educators to consider ways to ensure that this time is available. Furthermore, introducing supplementary content or tasks not required for course credit is more meaningful in the beginning rather than the middle or ending stages of a class group's developmental trajectory.

No primer on groups and how they work would be complete without considering the seemingly obvious point that a group is a collection of individuals. Group members each bring their own distinct needs to any collaboration in which they participate. In efforts to support interaction and collaboration among students, educators must bear in mind that each student is an individual learner as well as a member of a learning group.

Individual Support of Learners in Groups

Learning groups differ substantively from other groups in that the designated formal leader, the teacher, ultimately determines learners' grades. Given the critical importance of grades in higher education, working collaboratively and sharing the same grade can be perceived as threatening. During course activities when students work in groups, learners need continued assurance that the teacher will remain present and attentive to their needs as individuals.

If we empathize with students, we can easily appreciate how the threat of achieving poor grades or even failing might have a dramatic effect on their willingness to collaborate with fellow students in group projects. Abraham Maslow's (1982) well-known "hierarchy of needs" indicates that an individual's survival needs (physiological needs for air, water, and food, and safety needs for security and protection) must be fulfilled before the psychological needs for esteem, belonging, and self-actualization can be met. In the high stakes environment of higher education, learners need passing grades in order to survive. Given that students need to feel safe individually before they can be expected to engage in social activities such as belonging to a group, maintaining one-to-one communication with students takes on new significance. Simply sending regular private emails to each student, addressing students by name in written communication, and offering timely evaluative feedback on submissions can unobtrusively communicate the instructor's presence. This sense of presence provides learners with reassurance and feelings of security that are foundational to full group participation.

Group members have varying needs that their group can help satisfy (Beebe & Masterton, 2011). While some learners may have a high need for safety within a group, others may have a strong need for esteem and respect from the group. When specific individual needs are not met by the group, participants may dominate conversations, withdraw from participating, or introduce distractions. These dysfunctional behaviours slow the group's progression through the expected stages. Members may feel uncomfortable and dissatisfied with the collaborative process. Negative past experiences with groups can leave students reluctant to risk working together in future projects.

Online educators can play important roles in preventing negative group experiences. For example, intervening promptly and efficiently when the needs of an individual begin to interfere with a group's functioning is critical (Bergeron & Melrose, 2006). By monitoring collaborative work and requiring groups to attend to their own group process, teachers can remain well prepared to intervene when necessary. For instance, requiring groups to establish and submit their own "rules of engagement"—ground rules or guidelines—at the first meeting ensures that these will be available when needed. Contingency plans delineating consequences for not attending sessions, not submitting contributions, and not respecting members' time need to be clearly articulated in these group rules. Some groups may want group members to be graded individually. Others may wish to have input into the grades that their colleagues receive. Opportunities for progressive self-evaluation need to be built into the group's task timelines. The exercise of creating these rules, consequences, and self-evaluations, coupled with the formal requirement to submit a document that explains the rules, emphasizes the importance of group process in collaboration. In turn, this emphasis on process can communicate further assurance to students that they will be respected for their individual accountability during their involvement with collaborative work.

William Schutz's (1958) classic theory of interpersonal behaviour postulates that when individuals form and interact in groups, they all have needs for inclusion (feeling recognized and included, and reaching out to make others feel included), control (feeling in control, contesting issues, vying for leadership, and resolving conflicts), and affection (giving and receiving emotional support). Teaching actions that foster a sense of belonging, such as communicating that participation in group work is essential and ensuring that students are competent in the use of required tools such as the Internet and the learning management system, will begin to project a message that inclusion is important. Similarly, instructions phrased in a welcoming manner ("Let's make sure no one misses the chance to join a group") will invite students to pay attention to principles of inclusion.

Teaching actions such as allocating marks for participation, requiring group guidelines, and normalizing the experience of conflict as a natural part of a group's progress will help learners feel that they can maintain personal control during their experience as group members. The phrasing of instructions is important, as it models an underlying attitude. For example, "Reach out and let me know when things aren't going well" communicates that a designated formal leader (the teacher) is available and that group members will not be abandoned in managing issues they cannot resolve.

Teaching actions such as providing models of positive feedback during class discussions, writing genuinely encouraging comments on assignments, and affirming learner effort illustrate affection. Instructions such as "Showcase your leadership skills by offering help and encouragement when your group needs it most" communicate that offering emotional support is a valued behaviour in the class.

TEACHING ACTIVITIES AND STRATEGIES CONGRUENT WITH INSTRUCTIONAL IMMEDIACY THEORY

The strategies and interactive activities described below are affiliated with promoting instructional immediacy and can be adapted to a variety of online learning environments.

Projecting Immediacy

INTENTIONAL INTRODUCTIONS

Facilitating intentional introductions among members of a class is often overlooked as an important teaching activity. Student questions related to course content and the tasks that need to be done can dominate dialogue when students first meet one another in online courses. However, inviting students to thoughtfully introduce themselves has important implications for successful collaboration later. In groups of more than thirty learners, creating small subgroups for this introductory activity provides the opportunity for more meaningful in-depth initial sharing. Teachers who model a self-introduction that provides appropriate personal and professional information—including a photo, if desired—will establish an invitational tone. Such teacher introductions also role-model the appropriate level of self-disclosure. Identifying specific elements to include in the introduction—such as geographic location, employment, particular areas of interest within the course, time constraints, and hobbies and interests—provides the class with the opportunity to discover commonalities that facilitate connections and future conversations.

Another approach to facilitating introductions is to have students introduce each other. While this may work most efficiently in synchronous environments, it can be adapted to any learning experience. In face-to-face groups, dyads for introductions can be assigned by having students turn to the person sitting next to them. In online learning environments, dyads can be assigned by the teacher. Imposing a time limit and providing clear direction will keep the process moving smoothly. Usually, members of a dyad engage in private chat (either within the learning platform or using social media) and then introduce their partner to the remainder of the class. Modest learners may feel more comfortable sharing information with one classmate who listens attentively and asks probing questions than with introducing themselves directly to the entire class. Either way, introductions are the cornerstones for establishing further conversation.

While these further conversations are not generally expected to continue in the large class, actively suggesting that students connect with "even just one classmate" in the virtual class "coffee room" or by email will legitimize the notion that student-to-student interaction is important to course learning. Links to communication tools such as Skype or social media sites like Facebook and Twitter, and instructions for using them, can be included in the course syllabus. However, as Schutz (1958) emphasizes, when people become members of a group, they have high individual needs to feel included. Therefore, students who experience steep learning curves with technological programs that are new to them may not achieve connection with other learners. Rather, they may be left feeling frustrated, marginalized, and left behind before the formal learning even begins. It is important, therefore, that instructors assess learners to ensure that the learning activities are congruent with students' needs and abilities.

PUBLISH A "YEARBOOK"

After creating a forum within the course management system for students to post introductory messages, the instructor can continue to project immediacy by working with these messages. After teachers model an intentional introduction and invite students to introduce themselves, they compile all the postings and pictures (including their own) into a single document. This "yearbook," created and posted soon after all introductions have been posted, offers a glimpse into the life of each individual in the class and serves as handy reference as teacher and students get to know one another.

Publishing the yearbook can be as simple as cutting and pasting the postings and pictures into a word processing document and arranging them in alphabetical order. This gesture of working with the introductory information can subtly communicate to students that their teacher is present, attentive, and sincerely interested. Students can edit and add to their yearbook profiles throughout the course. The yearbook is kept within the course management system to protect students' privacy and maintain confidentiality.

EMBEDDING AUDIO AND VIDEO MESSAGES

Podcast messages from teachers can project immediacy. However, imagine the impact of "sharing the stage" by including the voices of students, present or past, in addition to the teacher's voice. Students who have already taken the class can compose brief audio and video messages that offer tips on completing course tasks. Melrose (2011) and Melrose and Swettenham (2013) collected audio messages of encouragement from senior students through digitally recorded telephone interviews. The messages were embedded in asynchronous self-directed introductory courses for health care professionals. Messages from past students included suggestions about time management, effective reading of textbooks, and communicating with instructors. As learners worked alone via distance, they were literally able to hear words of encouragement from students who had succeeded in the course.

Similarly, embedding video messages from the instructor or from experts in the area of study enhances immediacy. Students find it enlightening to see and hear descriptions of how course content is used. These videos can be solicited by the instructor and created specifically for the course, or students can seek out and share existing course-related videos. Descriptions of scenes from movies and television shows can be discussed when copyright restrictions prevent the inclusion of a popular film clip.

From the Field: Voiceover Feedback on Assignments

Diana Campbell gives voiceover feedback on assignments to provide students with meaningful comments. Providing feedback is essential to establishing positive teacher-student relationships. In online learning environments, particularly those dominated by text-based communication, hearing the voice of the teacher personalizes feedback. Voiceover feedback also offers an opportunity to project a tone of warmth and friendliness.

Diana tried this technique in one course and, based on positive student response, expanded it to other courses. After ensuring that students can open PDFs and have audio on their computers, she inserts a marking guide into the student's assignment and converts the entire Word document to PDF. Then she inserts the audio icon and records her oral feedback for the student.

From students' feedback, Diana has determined that this approach provides a greater sense of personal contact between student and instructor. She reports that this method allows her to provide more in-depth feedback in a time-efficient manner, and students have said that they enjoy being able to hear the tone of her comments.

Encouraging Group Collaboration

GROUP GUIDELINES

As discussed above, groups can be expected to progress through predictable stages, and individuals in a group may act in ways that either help or hinder that progression. The stakes are high in health care learning environments, and when students work in groups, their academic survival can be impacted by group dynamics. To support students toward success in any group project, instructors can require the submission of group guidelines or ground rules (written by the group) shortly after the group's first meeting. In addition, collaboration on grading group work can be encouraged when course syllabi can accommodate this. For example, the group could decide whether the same grade will be assigned to all members of the group and whether peer evaluation will be included.

As part of the process of creating group guidelines, a facilitated class discussion could give the students an opportunity to share positive "dreams" and negative "nightmares" that they have experienced in previous face-to-face or online class groups. Once the small working groups have been formed, members could be encouraged to link dreams to expectations and nightmares to consequences as they develop group guidelines. Since nightmares often occur when group members do not participate, consequences for not attending sessions or not submitting contributions must be clear in the consensus-based guidelines. Some groups may specify that a consequence of limited participation will be to seek help from the instructor, while others may agree that the member will be "fired" and the instructor notified of the group's decision. However varied group guidelines may be, having them in writing, agreed upon by all group members, and ready to use will help the group progress.

PEER EXEMPLARS

When students enter a learning space and begin to examine course materials, one of the first questions they grapple with is, What do I have to do? More precisely, students often wonder, What does the teacher want? Whether the class learning environment is a brick-and-mortar lecture hall, a multimedia online conference, or a solitary desk with an asynchronous self-directed learning module, students need to know what actions are required of them. One welcome supplement to well-written course study guides and assignment directions is a set of examples of work that other students in the course have done.

Copyright restrictions must be considered here. Some institutions will require stripping all identifying information from student products. Certainly, the students must be consulted and must grant their permission to have their work made available to others, and students posting their own work for others in the course to view can be reminded to remove private information such as student identification numbers. It is best to make example assignments created by former students available for only a short time and to stipulate that they are for illustrative purposes only and may not be reproduced. Most students find it very complimentary to be asked to share their work as exemplars.

Issues related to plagiarism can emerge when students have access to completed assignments. Posting examples of students' work is most suited to smaller classes where unique and personal adaptations of assignment guidelines are required. It is not suited to large introductory classes with assignments involving the broad collection of information or to assignments involving the description of a particular clinical condition. In these situations, the potential for plagiarism may outweigh the learning benefits. However, this practice is well suited to an assignment where health care students are asked to link their personal experiences to a specific situation or condition.

CREATING LEARNING PARTNERSHIPS

When faced with the task of sorting through new and seemingly overwhelming amounts of information, students can ease their anxiety by connecting with another learner in the same situation. In face-to-face learning experiences, particularly in the early stages of a course, health care students often gather during class coffee breaks and initiate such contacts. Online students lack these opportunities to connect physically, but teachers can create learning milieus that foster a similar connection. For example, learning partners can be assigned by pairing names in the order they appear on the class list or according to where students live. Alternatively, students can be invited to contact a classmate who might share a common interest, and if a learning partnership is formed, the names can be posted promptly for the rest of the class to see. In this way, the same individuals will not repeatedly be asked to partner, and all members of the group will be included. When the class does not have an even number of members, indicating that one partnership is expected to be a triad will model a commitment to inclusion within the class.

Learning partnerships do not necessarily have to be associated with formal assignments. Students can be invited to work with their partner on optional course activities such as puzzles or discussion questions. Some students may choose not to develop their learning partner relationship further, but encouraging partnerships implicitly communicates a class norm of connection among students. For example, virtual students may be encouraged to connect with classmates in an online forum established to mimic the coffee break experience. Simply setting up a coffee break forum, though, may not be sufficient to cultivate student-to-student connections. Instructors can invite students to connect with another student to clarify a question about expectations for the course. In some instances, such questions will be readily answered when the students collaborate. At other times, students will bring the question forward to the teacher. Either way, the confidence and connection that can accompany discussing a course matter with another individual involved with the same class facilitates the development of learning partnerships.

STUDY GROUPS

Another collaborative practice that teachers have found to be effective is the creation of study groups. This can be implemented by establishing an area within the course management system where students can indicate their interests, communicate their availability, and form groups to work together on their shared goals. Usually, students are not required to join a study group: membership is optional. However, teachers can encourage students to participate by posting scenarios about how this activity might strengthen learning or by inviting students to share anecdotes from previous learning experiences where study groups were helpful (or not helpful).

Although students are expected to organize their own study groups, teachers can offer to help with the process. For example, students can "register" their membership in a group with their teacher and submit reports on the group's activities. Teachers can also volunteer to attend selected study group sessions and pose questions intended to stimulate thinking and encourage students to reflect on what they are learning.

GROUP ASSIGNMENTS

Group assignments promote student-to-student connection and interaction. Describing group assignments in any course promotional material or institutional calendars cues students even before they join the class that group participation is expected and offers them the opportunity to begin thinking about their contribution.

The most effective group assignments entail incremental submissions. Early deadlines are best for the submission of group-determined participation guidelines (which also outline the consequences of not abiding by the guidelines). It is helpful to establish a private forum for each group where group members can meet to discuss their group processes and assignments. With the students' awareness, instructors can include themselves as a member of each private group forum.

Staying alert to any signs that a group is not progressing or is having issues that the group members cannot resolve internally allows the instructor to take action promptly. Opportunities for group members to earn credit for addressing group-maintenance functions can be built into the group project. For example, midway through the course, in the group's private working areas, group members can respond to questions such as, What is going well in your group right now?, What is one action that you have committed to that will improve group process?, or What are some approaches initiated by your fellow group members that have helped maintain group functionality? Similarly, once the group assignment is completed, group members can be encouraged to complete statements such as "One thing I appreciated about our group was . . ." or "One thing I would do differently next time is . . ." Providing wikis for both group tasks and group-maintenance functions in the private group forums will encourage ongoing dialogue about how the group is doing as well as what they are accomplishing in terms of their group goals.

ALUMNI AS A COURSE RESOURCE

Incorporating resources developed by former students into the course can illustrate the relevance and practical application of course material. Graduates or former students can be invited as guest speakers to present lectures or webinars based on their experiences with using course content in their professional practice. A program such as Adobe Connect can be used to record and archive these guest appearances, making them a permanent part of the course.

Course-related conversations between teachers and former students or practitioners can also be crafted into interactive resources. Posting an email from a graduate commenting on how an issue mentioned in class emerged in practice or linking to a practitioner's blog reflecting on a course topic injects real-world relevance into the course. When teachers extend this by eliciting comments from the class and organizing them to develop a response from the class as a whole, the conversation can develop in unanticipated and helpful directions. It is important to note that although posting email messages and links to blogs is useful, it is the teaching action of organizing a response from the class group that makes the activity interactive and collaborative. Personally connecting with and then "hearing back from" practitioners in learners' own field of study through these teacher-facilitated dialogues models professional conversations.

PEER EVALUATION

Peer evaluation activities can direct focus toward collaboration among students. Gathering peer feedback and factoring it into learners' final grades emphasizes engagement with others as important to success in the course. When an assignment calls for online presentations, it can include a requirement for evaluation questions related to their presentations. Programs like Survey Monkey are readily available to generate evaluation questionnaires that will ensure anonymous responses. However, class feedback about what audience members found most valuable, what they found less valuable, and what they suggest changing next time provides learners with a greater range of responses than just one teacher's feedback.

CONCLUSION

Teaching approaches that promote instructional immediacy and project a warm and friendly affect can enhance collaboration among learners. Teachers can project immediacy through choosing words that encourage connection and modelling the kind of communication that is expected from the students. This creates an engaging and invitational online learning environment in which learners feel recognized both as individuals and as members of a class group.

Theorists such as Bruce Tuckman, David Johnson, Frank Johnson, and Gilly Salmon offer important insight into the stages through which groups can be expected to progress. Appreciating how well-functioning groups work can guide instructors toward implementing the most effective teaching actions at the most opportune times in the group process. William Schutz's (1958) seminal work reminds us that when people join groups, they continue to have individual needs to be included, to feel in control, and to be received affectionately by others. When these individual needs interfere with a group's progress, teachers must intervene promptly. Maintaining one-to-one communication with students throughout their involvement with group work conveys instructional support and promotes accountability. Requiring groups to establish and then submit their group guidelines, their consequences for lack of adherence to the guidelines, and their plan for continually evaluating their group process and maintenance functions strengthens collaboration.

Teachers can project approachability and friendliness with diverse practices using a variety of technologies. They can encourage collaboration among students by implementing and adapting the ideas provided in this chapter or by creating their own activities designed to promote teamwork. With care and attention to communication among students and between the teacher and students, relationships within the class are bound to flourish as the course progresses, enhancing every aspect of learning.

REFERENCES

Andersen, J. F. (1979). Teacher immediacy as a predictor of teaching effectiveness. *Communication Yearbook, 3*, 543–559.

Anderson, T., Rourke, L., Archer, W., & Garrison, R. (2001). Assessing teaching presence in computer conferencing transcripts. *Journal of Asynchronous Learning Networks, 5*(2).

Arbaugh, J. B. (2001). How instructor immediacy behaviors affect student satisfaction and learning in Web-based courses. *Business Communication Quarterly, 64*(4), 42–54.

Baker, C. (2010). The impact of instructor immediacy and presence for online student affective learning, cognition, and motivation. *Journal of Educators Online, 7*(1). Retrieved from http://www.thejeo.com/Archives/Volume7Number1/BakerPaper.pdf

Baker, J. D. (2004). An investigation of relationships among instructor immediacy and affective and cognitive learning in the online classroom. *Internet and Higher Education, 7,* 1–13.

Beebe, S. A, & Masterson, J. T. (2011). *Communicating in small groups: Principles and practices* (10th ed.). Boston: Pearson.

Bergeron, K., & Melrose, S. (2006). Online graduate health care learners' perceptions of group work and helpful instructional behaviors. *Journal of Educational Technology, 3*(1), 74–80.

Christophel, D. M. (1990). The relationship among teacher immediacy behaviors, student motivation, and learning. *Communication Education, 39*(4), 323–340.

Christophel, D. M., & Gorham, J. (1995). A test-retest analysis of student motivation, teacher immediacy, and perceived sources of motivation and demotivation in college classes. *Communication Education, 44,* 292–306.

Gitin, E., Niemi, D., & Levin, J. (2012). Effects of online faculty immediacy behaviors on student performance. In *Proceedings of Global TIME 2012* (pp. 89–94), Association for the Advancement of Computing in Education (AACE).

Gorham, J. (1988). The relationship between verbal teacher immediacy behaviors and student learning. *Communication Education, 37*(1), 40–53.

Hess, J. A., & Smythe, M. J. (2001). Is teacher immediacy actually related to student cognitive learning? *Communication Studies, 52*(3), 197–219.

Hutchins, H. M. (2003). Instructional immediacy and the seven principles: Strategies for facilitating online courses. *Online Journal of Distance Learning Administration, 6*(3). Retrieved from http://www.westga.edu/~distance/ojdla/fall63/hutchins63.html

Jaques, D., & Salmon, G. (2007). *Learning in groups: A handbook for face-to-face and online environments* (4th ed.). London: Routledge.

Johnson, D. W., & Johnson, F. P. (1997). *Joining together: Group theory and group skills.* Boston: Allyn & Bacon.

Johnson, D. W., & Johnson, F. P. (2009). *Joining together: Group theory and group skills* (10th ed.). Upper Saddle River, NJ: Pearson Education.

Maslow, A. (1982). *Toward a psychology of being* (2nd ed.). Princeton, NJ: Van Nostrand.

Mehrabian, A. (1967). Attitudes inferred from nonimmediacy of verbal communication. *Journal of Verbal Learning and Verbal Behavior, 6,* 294–295.

Mehrabian, A. (1971). *Silent messages.* Belmont, CA: Wadsworth.

Melrose, S. (2009). Instructional immediacy online. In P. Rogers, G. Berg, J. Boettcher, C. Howard, L. Justice, & K. Schenk (Eds.), *Encyclopedia of Distance Learning* (2nd ed., Vol. 3, pp. P1212–1215). Hershey, PA: Information Science Reference.

Melrose, S. (2011). This worked for me! Podcast messages of encouragement from senior to junior students in an asynchronous self-paced online course. In *Proceedings of World Conference on E-Learning in Corporate, Government, Healthcare, and Higher Education 2011* (pp. 1486–1492). Chesapeake, VA: AACE.

Melrose, S., & Bergeron, K. (2006). Online healthcare graduate study learners' perceptions of instructional immediacy. *International Review of Research in Open and Distance Learning, 7*(1). Retrieved from http://www.irrodl.org/index.php/irrodl/article/viewArticle/255/477

Melrose, S., & Bergeron, K. (2007). Instructor immediacy strategies to facilitate group work in online graduate study. *Australasian Journal of Educational Technology, 23*(1), 132–148.

Melrose, S., & Swettenham, S. (2013). Asynchronous online peer assistance: Telephone messages of encouragement in post licensure nursing programs. *Journal of Peer Learning, 5*(1), 1–5.

Russo, T., & Benson, S. (2005). Learning with invisible others: Perceptions of online presence and their relationship to cognitive and affective learning. *Educational Technology and Society, 8*(1), 54–62. Retrieved from http://www.ifets.info/journals/8_1/8.pdf

Salmon, G. (2000). *E-moderating: The key to teaching and learning online.* London: Kogan Page.

Schutz, W. (1958). *The interpersonal underworld.* Palo Alto, CA: Science and Behavior Books.

Tuckman, B. (1965). Developmental sequence in small groups. *Psychological Bulletin, 63*(6), 384–399.

Tuckman, B., & Jensen, M. (1977). Stages of small group development. *Group and Organizational Studies, 2*(4), 419–427.

Walkem, K. (in press). Instructional immediacy in elearning. *Collegian: The Australian Journal of Nursing Practice, Scholarship, and Research.*

Wiener, M., & Mehrabian, A. (1968). *Language within language: Immediacy, a channel in verbal communication.* New York: Appleton-Century-Crofts.

Witt, P. L., Wheeless, L. R., & Allen, M. (2004). A meta-analytical review of the relationship between teacher immediacy and student learning. *Communication Monographs, 71*(2), 184–207.

Woods, R. H., & Baker, J. D. (2004). Interaction and immediacy in online learning. *International Review of Research in Open and Distance Learning, 5*(2). Retrieved from http://www.irrodl.org/index.php/irrodl/article/view/186/268

2

Invitational Theory: Developing the Plus Factor

Sue was a student in a fourth-year online course on nursing leadership. She had been an RN for many years and had recently decided to complete two years of online courses to obtain her bachelor's degree in nursing. Having been away from formal studies for many years, she was apprehensive about returning to school, despite being very competent in the workplace; in fact, her colleagues often asked her for help and advice, and she was often asked to preceptor new nurses. Yet she was nervous on September 1, the first day of the course.

Sue logged on early on day one, determined to make a positive impression on the instructor and her classmates. She was surprised that the instructor had already posted a warm, welcoming message and a photo of herself. The message seemed to be written just for

Sue—the words felt personal and the tone was encouraging and hopeful. *She looks really friendly and approachable*, Sue thought, making a mental note to ask the instructor questions about the course if she became confused or needed more information.

Proceeding to the first unit of the course, Sue found another surprise. The instructor had posted a short video outlining some of the key themes for the unit. The video was the first learning activity for the unit and had the intriguing title of "Me to You Video." Sue watched the video twice. The first time, she attended to the content, and the second time, she focused on the setting and on the teacher—what she was wearing, her smile, the surroundings of her office. Now knowing more about her teacher, she felt a little less nervous.

The course proceeded and Sue finished successfully, having learned a great deal about leadership and about her own leadership skills and abilities. Throughout the course, she had shared emails with her instructor, often asking for clarification or further information on a topic of interest. The instructor had responded to all of her queries promptly, and each response seemed personalized to Sue's issue. The words in the responses always addressed Sue's question and challenged her insights. Sue looked forward to these connections. Not once did she feel that she was "bothering" her instructor.

Although Sue relished her success in the course, she admitted to her husband that she would miss the class. Beyond the interactions with the instructor, she had forged many positive relationships with other students in the course. The learning environment in this online course encouraged students to work collaboratively and to share their knowledge, skills, and ideas with one another generously. Through these interactions, the students got to know one another. The online "coffee forum" was especially busy in this class. Sue felt inspired to continue on in her studies.

BACKGROUND THEORY

What Is Invitational Theory?

The teaching approach and techniques that Sue's instructor used was based on invitational theory, a model of professional practice developed by William Watson Purkey. Purkey (1992) used the word *invitational* to mean offering something valuable and summoning cordially. An invitation is an intentional and caring act of communication designed to offer something beneficial for consideration. "In invitational theory, everybody and everything adds to, or subtracts from, human existence. Ideally, the factors of people, places, policies, programs, and processes should be so intentionally inviting as to create a world where each individual is cordially summoned to develop physically, intellectually, and emotionally" (Purkey, 1992, p. 12). The foundation of invitational theory is the belief that one person can be of benefit to others; in the educational context, this benefit usually accrues through an invitation to participate in the learning environment (Purkey & Novak, 1996). However, it is always the choice of the individual (the student) to accept or reject the invitation (Riner, 2010).

The core assumption of invitational theory is that the learning environment affects students' learning (Haigh, 2008). People, places, policies, programs, and processes, the five pillars upon which pedagogy is constructed, provide a framework for assessing inviting practices (Haigh, 2011; Schmidt, 2007). Manipulating these pillars, according to Riner (2010), potentially influences student success. In 2010, Shaw and Siegel created invitational theory and practice (ITP), which combines various aspects and elements of invitational theory to create a comprehensive framework. Schmidt (2007) notes that "invitational education" is essentially an inclusive model of communication and human relations.

Foundations of Invitational Theory

DEMOCRACY

Purkey and Novak (2008) explain that democracy is a social ideal founded on a belief that people are important, that they have potential to evolve, and that self-governance is appropriate. Democracy in education includes purposeful dialogue, mutual respect, and participation in shared activities. In other words, in a democratic learning environment, individuals work together to co-create the ethical character and social practices of the learning milieu and learners are involved in decisions that affect them. Participants act responsibly. Teachers "do with" rather than "do to" students. For example, rather than talk about a teacher "empowering" students, which implies a "doing to" approach in which the teacher performs an action directed at students (the power resides with the teacher, who then bestows it on students), invitational theory uses the neutral noun *empowerment* (Schmidt, 2007). A democratic class is one in which student innovation and creativity is valued and encouraged and learning is a shared experience.

Schmidt (2007) emphasizes the role that encouragement plays in a democratic environment. Encouragement aligns with the fundamental philosophy of "being with" rather than "doing to" (p. 20). According to Schmidt, praise is not the same as encouragement: while praise is somewhat superficial and produces short-term effects, encouragement comes from a genuine commitment or authenticity and produces long-lasting results.

PERCEPTION

Invitational theory is rooted in the belief that student behaviour is determined by student perception. Because our view of the world influences our behaviour, that view is our blueprint for action.

Through our perceptions (based on our experiences and knowledge), we draw conclusions and make decisions (Schmidt, 2007). We develop our views based on present and past experiences (Purkey & Novak, 2008). Schmidt (2007) emphasizes that the invitational approach "embraces, celebrates, and honors diversity" in the educational milieu, since everyone's perceptions are unique (p. 16).

SELF-CONCEPT

Self-concept, the beliefs that individuals hold about themselves, influences behaviour and capacity (Purkey & Novak, 2008). Since invitational theory proposes that positive self-concept is vital to successful learning (Riner, 2003), invitational approaches focus on helping students to enhance their self-concept. Teachers who practice from an invitational theory stance, realizing that the self-concept is fragile, behave "gently, appropriately, and with great care when asking others to change course, accept challenges, learn new information, and make positive contributions to the larger group" (Schmidt, 2007, p. 21).

Assumptions of Invitational Theory

Three basic interdependent assumptions underlie invitational theory. First, invitational theory assumes that students are able, valuable, and capable of self-direction, and should be treated accordingly (Purkey, 1992, p. 5). Second, process is as important as the outcome or product. Cooperative and collaborative alliances in learning environments are important elements of process. Third, humans possess untapped potential, and educational programs should be intentionally designed to help people reach this potential (Purkey & Novak, 2008).

The Four Central Values of Invitational Theory

The values that invitational theory embraces are trust, respect, optimism, and intentionality in the educational environment (Purkey, 1992). *Trust* includes reliability, consistency, dependability, personal authenticity, and truthfulness in the thoughts, behaviours, and beliefs of participants in the educational community (Purkey & Novak, 2008). In a trusting relationship, participants recognize each other as interdependent and as the authorities on their own best way of being and becoming.

Respect is based on the recognition that people are able, valuable, and responsible, and that people should be treated as such. An invitational environment is respectful when this is acknowledged. Respect is closely linked with the value of care, which, in this context, is concern expressed warmly for the well-being of others (Shaw & Siegel, 2010, p. 108). Respect is made manifest in the acknowledgement of each individual's independence of thought (Riner, 2010). Invitational educational approaches do not use coercion.

According to Purkey (1992), *optimism* is a chosen perspective or outlook on the world and on people and is based on the underlying goal of positive outcomes. Optimism is based on the assumption that human potential has no limits.

Finally, *intentionality* means that teachers deliberately create and offer invitational environments (Purkey, 1992). An invitational educational milieu is created when optimism, trust, and respect (which includes care) are intentionally cultivated. These essential values of invitational theory—trust, respect, optimism, and intentionality—offer a means through which humans can create and maintain optimally inviting learning environments.

Ways of Functioning in Invitational Theory

According to invitational theory, instructors can function in four different modes: intentionally inviting, intentionally disinviting, unintentionally inviting, or unintentionally disinviting. Educators can unintentionally create disinviting environments by inadvertently exhibiting a lack of trust, respect, and optimism. Conversely, environments can be unintentionally inviting when trust, respect, optimism, and intentionality are serendipitously present, rather than being consciously created. When instructors function in an intentionally inviting manner, they consistently and purposefully exhibit the four central values of invitational theory, whereas when those values are deliberately withheld, the result is an intentionally disinviting atmosphere.

INTENTIONALLY INVITING

Teachers and course designers can generally create effective educational environments by being intentionally inviting. According to Purkey (1992), intentionally inviting educators treat learners as individuals, develop trust through honesty in interactions, behave ethically, maintain an optimistic perspective, sustain energy and enthusiasm, and keep high expectations. Purkey concludes that invitational theory "carries the basic message that human potential, while not always evident, is always there, waiting to be discovered and invited forth" (1992, p. 15). Purkey and Novak (2008) argue that invitational approaches in education "significantly increase" this human potential.

Research has demonstrated that inviting educational environments have positive implications for learners. Cook (2005) found that when clinical nursing faculty intentionally created an invitational milieu, student anxiety decreased. By using invitational theory to create what they called "invitational education," Stanley, Juhnke, and Purkey (2004) were able to enhance school culture, improve academic achievement, and help stakeholders view concerns as symptoms rather than causes. In another study (Hunter and Smith, 2007), invitational education was applied to high school art classes, resulting in a more positive learning environment for students and teachers. Chant, Moes, and Ross (2009) found that including the collaborative processes of invitational theory encouraged teacher creativity, and Thompson (2004) concluded that employing the philosophy of invitational education created a more welcoming climate. Paxton (2003) advocates the use of invitational theory principles in e-learning, noting that e-learning will only succeed if educators intentionally create environments that preserve dignity and encourage communication.

UNINTENTIONALLY DISINVITING

In unintentionally disinviting learning situations, accidental or unplanned behaviours can result in a less positive environment and limit learners' potential and positive outcomes. For example, using an online environment to "throw information" at students with no opportunities for student interaction can be experienced as deeply disinviting (Paxton, 2003, p. 923). Paxton (2003) identifies some of the more common disinviting practices currently experienced by learners who are new to the e-learning environment and suggests practical ways in which online educators can make the environment more invitational. Some of these practices are an overwhelming amount of course material, learning activities that are irrelevant to the learning needs of the students, learning that occurs in isolation, one-way delivery of course content, and absence of opportunities for students to interact with one another and with the instructor regarding course materials.

UNINTENTIONALLY INVITING

According to invitational theory, teachers may exhibit behaviours or create courses that students find inviting without deliberately setting out to do so, thus being unintentionally inviting (Shaw & Siegel, 2010). This can result in positive outcomes for both students and instructors; however, instructors may be left wondering why this occurred. Upon reflection, they may recognize possible reasons for success (such as behaviours that helped create an invitational milieu) and then use this knowledge to become intentionally inviting in future course offerings.

INTENTIONALLY DISINVITING

Intentionally disinviting learning situations are characterized by deliberate behaviours that seek to injure or disrupt positive outcomes of a learning experience and the potential of participants (Shaw & Siegel, 2010). This has possible negative consequences for all involved.

It follows that inviting or disinviting behaviours (whether intentional or not) can have two outcomes: "beneficial presence or lethal presence" (Shaw & Siegel, 2010, p. 109). Educators who adopt what Purkey (1992) calls an "inviting stance" employ behaviours and approaches that result in positive outcomes, An educator with an inviting stance understands and enacts the foundations, values, and assumptions that underpin invitational theory.

In summary, invitational theory (or invitational theory and practice) is a useful way to examine and understand how people, places, policies, processes, and programs influence positive outcomes in educational environments. At its best, invitational practice becomes invisible (Shaw & Siegel, 2010): that is, skilled practitioners of invitational theory integrate this inviting way of thinking and being so that it just becomes part of who they are. Inviting educators confront all situations (including difficult ones) with invitational attitudes and behaviours and, in doing so, have a positive and constructive approach to teaching. Shaw and Siegel (2010) call this "the plus factor." Invitational theory provides online teachers and course designers with insight regarding elements that may enhance positive student outcomes. Finally, Purkey reminds us that the learning should be enjoyed. Educators who subscribe to invitational theory look for opportunities to celebrate, enjoy others, and find good cheer. As Purkey writes, "How easy it is to overlook life's joys" (2006, p. 99). Invitational theory gives us permission—in fact, it requires us—to seek the delight in teaching and learning.

TEACHING ACTIVITIES AND STRATEGIES CONGRUENT WITH INVITATIONAL THEORY

This section describes practical teaching activities and techniques that online educators can use in course design and instruction to create more invitational educational environments. These practices are organized according to the values that underlie invitational theory—trust, respect, optimism, and intentionality.

Developing Trust

Trust is important in developing effective interpersonal relationships among students in online classes (Wade, Cameron, Morgan, & Williams, 2011). While trust is often described as essential to positive relationships, a common understanding of trust is elusive. We view trust as a multifaceted, fragile, emotional, interpersonal phenomenon that is fundamental to human interaction (Andrei, Oţoiu, Isailă, & Băban, 2010). Trust is dynamic: not only does it provide a basis for a relationship, but it is also shaped by the relationship (Nooteboom, 2006).

Trust develops over time. As an online course progresses, members of the class (students and instructor) become known to one another. If participants discover commonalities and develop positive regard for one another, they may begin to trust. Trust also develops when groups work on tasks that create interdependence (Andrei et al., 2010). Some teaching activities have the development of trust as a primary goal. With others, the development of trust is a corollary outcome. Teaching practices that may have a positive influence on trust in the online classroom are described in detail below, and instructors are encouraged to adapt these practices according to their students' needs and interests.

"ME TO YOU" YOUTUBE VIDEOS

When we teach in face-to-face classrooms, we have the opportunity in each class to greet the students, offer them a short update regarding how we see the class progressing, give a brief overview of key points covered in the last class, and perhaps offer a word of encouragement. Online teachers can achieve a similar effect with "Me to You" videos.

As the name suggests, "Me to You" videos are personalized for each class. The "me" is the course instructor and the "you" is the members of that particular section of the course. Because the videos are unique to each offering of a course, they need to be prepared by (and feature the face of) the course teacher. Optimally, a new video is offered at the start of each unit of a course. Furthermore, if the videos are made "fresh" each time a course is offered, the instructor can personalize the message for that specific group of learners.

To be most effective, the videos are largely unscripted: that is, the instructor just chats to the class in an informal voice, preferably with a warm and inviting conversational tone. Since part of the goal of this strategy is to have the instructor seem real to the learners, it is effective to create the videos in the teacher's office space, the physical place where he or she may be interacting with students online. One professor sits in her home office to record her videos; in the background, students see a wall of textbooks, family photos, and other personal effects. When these videos are shared throughout the course, they become concrete evidence that the instructor is participating in the course. "Me to You" videos may help to enhance the feeling that the instructor is engaged with students in their learning journey and to mitigate the sense of isolation that students tend to feel in online courses (Revere & Kovach, 2011).

Through the visual and auditory contact of "Me to You" videos, the instructor becomes known to the learners. Nonverbal clues to the instructor's personality may become evident, and some of the instructor's personal life (hobbies, family, values) may be shared appropriately through what the students see on the screen. The students thus get to know more about the instructor, which facilitates the development of trust, a foundation for the invitational classroom.

Making and sharing a YouTube video is as easy as sitting in front of a webcam and pressing record. Information about this process is available online: see, for example, http://www.youTube.com/t/creators_ corner or http://www.ehow.com/how_2036208_youtube-video.html.

The "Me to You" videos are short, about two minutes in length. They are greetings, not lectures. The first video in a course may be the most important, since students will make an instant assessment based on first impressions. A genuinely engaging welcome from the instructor can help create a convivial atmosphere. If the initial "Me to You" video is awaiting learners when they first log in to their course, it can be the first step toward an invitational environment and the establishment of trust.

From the Field: A Warm Introduction with a Personal Touch

Carol Anderson writes a warm, personalized introductory email to each student to help establish trust in the student-instructor relationship. Beginning with students' names, she welcomes them and outlines her expectations of them and what they can expect from her as their instructor. She also lets them know the best time to contact her. She is always available during the specified time and responds quickly to emails to help build trust.

Carol includes comments about the makeup of the class to give students some idea of who is participating in the course and to paint a picture of the group: for example, she may describe the age range, geographical distribution, and academic experience of the students. She also includes her own profile in an attachment. Her introduction sets the tone for the upcoming interactions.

Generally, students have provided very positive feedback about Carol's introduction. One student wrote, "The instructor set the tone for the course in her introduction. Expectations and ground rules were set out." Another said, "Carol's initial comments made a significant impression upon me. They set the stage for an open, approachable and supportive environment that continued to grow." And yet another described Carol as being "extremely professional" and as having "a sense of warmth" and a "great virtual presence."

PHOTOVOICE

Photovoice allows course participants to share their values, biases, hobbies, interests, and personalities with the class. In doing so, they become better known to one another, enabling the development of trust within the class community.

Photovoice originated as a participatory action research method. Specifically, Wang and Burris (1997) used photographs to elicit responses from study participants on issues related to their health and community needs. Through this research method, participants, regardless of their literacy levels, were enabled to reflect and effectively communicate their perceptions and insights (Wang, 1999).

Perry (2006) transformed the photovoice research method into an online teaching technique. The instructor posts a different digital photographic image at the beginning of each unit of an online course. Each purposefully selected image is accompanied by a reflective question. Students are encouraged to view the photograph, consider the question, and contribute to an online discussion forum provided for each photovoice activity. The photovoice activity is optional and ungraded. Figure 1 offers an example of a photovoice activity used in a course on organizational change.

Students' photovoice responses often reveal something about them that may not be as easily shared in traditional discussion forums. For example, in responding to the photovoice shown in figure 1, one student, noticing the garden in the photo, commented as part of her response that her hobby was gardening. Others in the class shared this interest and connections were established around this hobby. The "coffee forum" (a forum established for informal conversations unrelated to the course) became very active as this subgroup of the class exchanged gardening tips. Eventually, these students formed a working group and made an excellent presentation to the class on a course theme. Their shared interest, discovered through the photovoice activity, may have helped to establish trust among group members, thereby preparing them to work together effectively as a team on course work.

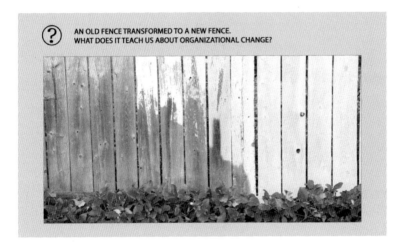

AN OLD FENCE TRANSFORMED TO A NEW FENCE.
WHAT DOES IT TEACH US ABOUT ORGANIZATIONAL CHANGE?

Figure 1. Example of a photovoice.

Photovoice also provides a means by which instructor presence is established and maintained throughout a course. If the photovoice images and questions are provided at the beginning of each unit, students may log on to the course regularly to see what new image has been posted. In a study of the effect of photovoice on student engagement, one student commented, "I couldn't wait to see what would be revealed behind that virtual paperclip," referring to the digital image and reflective question that awaited the class each week (Perry & Edwards, 2010). Furthermore, since the instructor chooses and shares the images, the themes portrayed disclose something about the teacher. For example, in the same study by Perry and Edwards (2010), one student noted, "Looking at the images was like visiting the professor's home . . . it was like looking through the professor's art collection." This student came to know through the photovoice images that the professor liked nature, enjoyed gardening, and had a fondness for flowers. The student noted that this experience made the professor "real" to her in a virtual world. When course participants become more real to one another, trust may develop more easily.

As a variation on the photovoice activity, students could take on the role of choosing and posting the photovoice images and reflective questions. This would give them the opportunity to share their own photographs and would encourage them to get to know the topic well enough to develop a meaningful reflective question.

From the Field: Photovoice in a Qualitative Research Course

Sharon Moore uses a variation of photovoice in her advanced qualitative research course. To introduce each topic in the course, she combines a photograph with a quotation to tie the image to the concept on which she is focusing. The image is used as a visual introduction to the unit of study.

For example, the first unit of the research methods course that Sharon designed begins with a photograph of a path accompanied by a quotation by Tsukiyama (1994) that reads: "Even if you walk the same path a hundred times, you will see something new each time." The text of the study guide refers to the fact that although students may have studied qualitative approaches in the past, this course will encourage them to go deeper in their understanding of why one particular methodology might be chosen over another one.

For example, the first unit of the research methods course that Sharon designed begins with a photograph of a path accompanied by a quotation by Tsukiyama

(1994) that reads: "Even if you walk the same path a hundred times, you will see something new each time." The text of the study guide refers to the fact that although students may have studied qualitative approaches in the past, this course will encourage them to go deeper in their understanding of why one particular methodology might be chosen over another one.
Sharon uses this teaching technique to link an artistic pedagogical tool to a concept. The photograph appeals to a different sense and adds another component to an online print-based course.

GROUP PROJECTS: CRACKER BARREL COLLABORATIONS

As noted earlier, trust may develop as class participants work together interdependently on a task or project. The nature of the group project will vary depending on the topic, group responsibilities, products required, number of group members, and selection process for forming groups. To effectively promote trust, the group project needs to be challenging, require contributions from all group members, and have a collaborative or interdependent element required for success. The Cracker Barrel group project meets these requirements.

The activity takes its name from the cracker barrels found in old country stores, around which customers used to gather and chat. In a Cracker Barrel session, a group of about five students (assigned to the group by the instructor) make a 15-minute presentation on a key issue or question about a course topic using a meeting platform such as Adobe Connect. (Sessions may be audio only or use video as well, depending on the technological options available.) Following the presentation, the group members lead a 30-minute roundtable discussion on the topic with the entire class. Sessions occur in real time but can be recorded for those who cannot be present at the scheduled time.

Students in each group collaborate to prepare the presentation and to lead the roundtable discussion on the topic. The scoring rubric gives credit for evidence that all members of the group participated in both of these aspects of the Cracker Barrel session. As a follow-up to this activity, students may be asked to write a brief paper (about two pages, double-spaced) in which they reflect on the collaborative processes used by the group and on what they learned about collaboration. The reflection paper may include references to related theory.

Promoting Respect

Literature related to effective teaching, including effective online instruction, frequently mentions the importance of respect. Participants in the online educational milieu (teachers and students) need to treat one another with respect if effective relationships are to develop and optimal learning is to occur. Respect is more than "nice to have." Respect is essential for establishing an invitational learning environment.

As Cohen (2001) points out, respect is a sentiment that one person has with regard to another: it implies two people. Palmer-Jones and Hoertdoerfer (2008, p. 3) argues that respect is "both a way of *behaving* and a way of *feeling*," one that implies "consideration," that is, the action of taking the other person's feelings into account, and "esteem," that is, an emotional orientation. These authors all note that respect is often a mutual and reciprocal experience. Frijda (1986) summarizes respectful action as "treating others as you want to be treated."

A RESPECTFUL COMMUNICATION STYLE

Respect begins with the very first communiqué that the instructor shares with the class or with a student. The beginning seeds of respect, which will potentially blossom into a mutually respectful relationship, are carried in the tone, structure, content, and word choice of the instructor's first posting or email. For example, does the email or posting begin with a greeting? An effective face-to-face teacher entering a physical classroom on day one would not launch into instructions regarding the course without first giving a friendly greeting or welcome. Respectful emails and postings that are perceived as invitational have both a warm greeting and a parting phrase such as "over to you" or "all the best." These salutations demonstrate and engender respect in the online learning milieu.

The language used in online correspondence is also important in communicating respect for students. Messages that are positive, use inclusive language, and are shared with an appropriate audience all communicate respect. With regard to positive language, some words have a more uplifting feeling than others. For example, "I would be delighted" sounds more enthusiastic and positive than "Okay, I will do that." The instruction "Glance through the article to find ideas that are relevant to your experience" is more encouraging than "Read the article." Using inclusive language also connotes respect: using "we," for example, includes the teacher in the learning community. Careful word choices can make typed words (and the online teacher) come alive to students and can help ensure that the humanness of online messaging is not lost. In part, this is achieved through using words that convey emotions such as caring, compassion, concern, joy, excitement, or interest.

Taking care to send messages through appropriate channels and to the right audiences demonstrates an awareness of how others would like to be treated. For example, feedback specific to a student should be shared though private communication channels to avoid causing the student any public embarrassment. This thoughtful and careful direction of messages is another sign of respect that online instructors can role-model through their communication style and techniques.

JOIN A COMMUNITY OF PRACTICE

A community of practice (CoP) is a group of individuals who share a concern, interest, or passion and who interact regularly with a focus on this commonality. A CoP is made up of three components: the domain, the community, and the practice (Wenger, 1998). Examples of CoPs include a group of painters seeking new forms of expression, a group of scientists working on a similar problem, and a group of first-year nurses helping each other to cope with the stresses of academic life.

A simple effective learning activity involves inviting students to seek out a CoP that relates to their professional interests. Students join this CoP, participate over several weeks, and then share their experiences and reflections with their classmates in a conference forum.

The CoP learning activity accomplishes several learning outcomes. Students discover and become involved in CoPs that might be helpful to them during and after the course. In order to share their experiences with their classmates, students need to reflect on their experiences in the CoP and consolidate their thoughts into a succinct posting, thus gaining experience communicating online with others who share their interests.

The CoP learning activity helps to build respect in the online learning environment, in part because students are exposed to diverse opinions expressed in the CoP. This exposure to others who have similar interests but bring different perspectives to the larger discussion develops awareness of the synergy that can result from variety. When students share their reflections with their class, this observation is often expressed as part of the insight they gain from this learning activity.

As a variation on the CoP activity, students can join a discussion blog on a topic of professional interest. The instructor can encourage students to discover a relevant blog on their own or can direct them to a specific blog. One advantage to having all students join the same blog is that their individual reflections posted on the course forum will be based on common experiences.

Enhancing Optimism

People often choose to cultivate an optimistic outlook because they believe it will lead to positive outcomes. According to Purkey (1992), optimistic individuals embrace the belief that human potential is limitless. The invitational education environment depends on the optimism of the teacher and on the development of optimistic attitudes in students. The teacher is often the catalyst for enhancing a tone of optimism in the classroom and for the development of optimistic attitudes. Some online learning activities may aid the teacher in this goal.

MOMENT AT THE MOVIES

For this activity, the teacher provides students with links to clips from inspiring movies related to the course content. For example, in a course on effective education, excerpts from movies such as *Dead Poets Society* or *Mr. Holland's Opus* or from television series such as *Glee* can be used to illustrate exemplary educators who inspire optimism in others. Students watch the clips and share their observations in response to a specific reflection question (provided by the teacher) in an online discussion forum. The reflection question can be as simple as "How did X inspire students?" Often students bring in their own examples of movies or television shows that they found inspiring, furthering the breadth and depth of the discussion.

Other course topics will require different movie or television clips. These examples are easily located. For example, searching the Internet for "movies about nurses" provides a list of movies with insights and themes useful to nursing students, including *MASH*, *Florence Nightingale*, *Miss Evers' Boys*, and *Wit*.

The "Moment at the Movie" learning activity usually results in a class discussion in which students express pride in their chosen profession and indicate that they are inspired to excel in their field. Furthermore, the tone of the discussion is optimistic: that is, they can and will succeed.

MUSIC

Because music can be a source of inspiration, using music in online teaching is another way to increase the optimism felt by the class community. One of the many ways to include music in an online course is choosing a theme song. This "anthem" can be linked into the course at strategic points such as the beginning and end of the course as a whole, at the beginning of units or major sections, or at particularly stressful moments such as an assignment deadline or an exam. Not all learners will find music inspiring, but the link to the course theme song provides students with the option to play the song if they find it helpful.

Choosing appropriate music is essential to success of this strategy. Often, an instrumental selection is best, since lyrics can be distracting and can also be misinterpreted. The tone and tempo of the selection needs to be spirited and engaging without being too aggressive. The fact that people often have powerful emotional responses to music is what makes this an effective strategy, but it also opens up the possibility of a negative response. For example, a tune that most people find positive and uplifting might trigger memories of a death or a break-up in a few individuals. The trick is to find a musical selection that is fairly neutral but stops short of being insipid "elevator" music, and this requires skill on the part of the teacher. The instructor in a class on teacher education used "Destiny," an instrumental piece from Peter Kind's album *The Fallen Angel* (available at https://www.jamendo.com/en/track/1001530/destiny). With its sprightly, uplifting beat, it inspired feelings of optimism in most of the class participants.

There are also copyright issues to consider when using music in online courses. Copyright administrators at an instructor's institution can help to ensure that protocol is not breached. Although many online music sources, such as jamando.com, state that they are copyright and royalty free, copyright issues may still exist and the necessary steps must be taken to ensure that the music is being used appropriately.

Students can be encouraged to select the course music through group consensus, or individual students can choose the course music for one unit or section of the course. Consensus decision making encourages team building and effective conflict resolution. When individual students contribute music selections, they have the opportunity to share something about themselves with the group: their choices often come with a story or background explanation, which facilitates community building. Both variations have pedagogical advantages.

Another way to include music in an online course is to encourage students to listen to baroque music while studying and writing their reflections or scholarly papers. Instructors can provide links to online baroque music such as http://www.youtube.com/watch?v=mURZQNpKiLQ or http://www.youtube.com/watch?v=CVAcLaNGZv4. Research demonstrates that listening to baroque music while studying can enhance learning and concentration (Esman, 2011). This is, in part, attributed to the lively and engaging quality of baroque music, which is experienced by many as uplifting. Music that is carefully chosen, offered as an option rather than an imposition, and skillfully integrated into an online course can fuel a sense of optimism in the class community.

CARTOON ANALYSIS

Often referred to colloquially as "the best medicine," laughter lifts us up and energizes individuals and groups. Although this applies to online courses as well, sharing laughter and humour online can be a challenge, especially if only written methods are used. Using video in online classes adds to the effectiveness of humour because nonverbal cues are often essential to humour. Online instructors can take deliberate steps to integrate humour into courses in order to raise the optimism of the group. One way to do this is to use cartoon analysis.

For this activity, students are asked to seek out cartoons on a course topic, keeping in mind that valuable lessons can often be found in cartoon humour. Teachers can provide students with current links to cartoon sites as a starting point. After they find a course-related cartoon that appeals to their sense of humour, they text or email another class member to share their cartoon and explain what they learned from it. This helps to develop relationships between students in the course. As a variation, the students' sharing can be done in a course forum for all the class to see and respond to.

Demonstrate Caring

In invitational learning environments, learners sense that the instructor views each person as a valued member of the community of learners. Students feel that the instructor has a genuine interest in them. This is demonstrated by the instructor's willingness to provide them with individualized feedback and personalized learning opportunities. In part, invitational instructors show that they care about students by being present in the online course, providing frequent posts, responding promptly to student questions, giving substantive feedback on postings and assignments, and distributing and returning assignments in a timely manner. In addition to these basic approaches, the techniques that follow demonstrate an instructor's care and might be incorporated into online courses.

From the Field: Being There!

Joyce Springate uses an online teaching approach that she calls "Being there!" Joyce wants students to know that she believes in their abilities and their desire to complete the program, so she tries to "hear" what they are asking or saying in each posting. She responds to their concerns as quickly as possible. If the postings are well done, Joyce gives personalized feedback that will encourage more of the same. If students are having difficulties related to health, family, or work, Joyce does whatever she can to help and encourage them. She usually offers an extension to give students some deadline flexibility when they are facing extreme stressors. While Joyce keeps her responses and messages to students as short and clear as possible, she expresses compassion and patience in her communiqués with students to minimize misunderstandings and to convey her care about them and their learning.

REFLECTIVE OR PARALLEL POETRY

Emotion is difficult to convey online, but poems provide a vehicle for sharing feelings within the limitation of words. Reflective or parallel poetry is useful as a teaching tool both in helping students to achieve learning outcomes in the affective domain that may involve a change in attitudes or beliefs and in helping learners and instructors to express feelings and emotional experiences.

In parallel poetry, the instructor provides an example poem on a topic related to the course content. Haikus, odes, limericks, and narrative and couplet poems have been used successfully for this artistic pedagogical technology. The example poem is usually written by the instructor, although a published poem can be used if its theme corresponds with the course content. Students are invited to create their own poem (a parallel poem) after reading the example poem. The poem written by the student is to parallel the structure of the demonstration poem and reflect a specified course theme. The following is an example of a teacher-constructed poem and a student's parallel poem on the topic of caring.

Teacher Poem

> *On Caring . . .*
>
> It is difficult
> To put into precise words,
> What it means to care.
> Is it giving, not taking?
> Is it listening, not talking?
> Is it bending, not standing strong?

Student Poem

> *On Caring . . .*
>
> What does it mean to care?
> It is giving and taking, at just the right moments.
> It is listening and talking, in perfect balance.
> It is bending and standing strong, strong enough
> for two.

Poems are effective teaching strategies in part because writers need to understand a topic in order to write a poem about it. According to van Manen (1990), poetry is the perfect medium for giving voice to abstract and complex topics such as human interaction. Additional examples of such topics are compassion, human connection, motivation, inspiration, and caring, topics that are often part of nursing and other human services curricula. As van Manen (1990) notes, poems help to expose the tacit and unspoken within the limitation of words. Poems have the potential to communicate the essence of topics that are difficult to write about, including personal beliefs, values, and philosophies.

Since the poem that is to be paralleled by the students is written or chosen by the instructor, it gives learners insight into that instructor's values, priorities, and attitudes. In this way, the parallel poetry activity is also a technique through which instructors share themselves with students. It offers the opportunity for students to come to know their instructor as a caring, compassionate person.

PHOTOSTORIES AND AUDIO CASTS

Opportunities for students to get to know their online instructors are often limited. Although a photo of an instructor may accompany each posting in a course forum, the teacher may not become as animated and real to learners as face-to-face instructors are. In order to create an invitational educational milieu, it is important for online teachers to find ways to disclose appropriate personality attributes and personal details to learners to reveal that they are caring individuals. In face-to-face teaching, students hear the instructor's voice, see how instructors dress and present themselves, and often hear personal details integrated into class discussions or during shared breaks. All of these experiences help learners to know their teachers at an appropriate personal level. To achieve this level of intimacy online, teachers can use self-disclosure through a photostory or an audio cast.

A photostory, which is a combination of images and voice, can be created using PowerPoint with voiceover narration or other open-source software programs. The most important consideration in creating a photostory is to include images of the instructor and of activities or topics of interest to him or her. The voice on the photostory is that of the instructor. An effective photostory is short (less than five minutes) and is generally posted early in the course. It can be accompanied by a written posting conveying that it is being provided as an opportunity for students to get to know the instructor in a more personal way.

A variation on the photostory is an audio cast in which instructors record a short biography for the students using a friendly, informal tone. The instructor provides some interesting details about his or her interest and expertise in the course topic and welcomes students to the course. Like the photostory, the audio cast is uploaded near the beginning of the course as part of the instructor's welcome.

Demonstrating Intentionality

In order to facilitate effective learning, online instructors need to deliberately create an invitational environment: that is, an educational environment that is perceived as optimistic and rooted in a sense of trust, respect, and caring. Using any of the teaching techniques outlined in this chapter can demonstrate that the instructor believes in the importance of an invitational environment is taking action to create such a learning environment. The key message is this—an invitational learning environment requires deliberate intervention on the part of the online instructor. While a disinviting learning environment can occur without teacher intervention, an inviting learning environment requires an ongoing cycle of assessment, planning, intervention, and evaluation of the learners, learning needs, and effectiveness of teaching strategies throughout the duration of the course.

CONCLUSION

Instructors with an invitational attitude, an interest in creating an online learning environment that students perceive as invitational, and a willingness to deliberately choose teaching strategies and techniques that facilitate this experience may have "the plus factor" (Shaw & Siegel, 2010). The plus factor attitude and approach to online teaching can have important benefits for learners: they may be more engaged in the learning experience and achieve learning outcomes more successfully. The first step in becoming a plus factor online educator is gaining an awareness of invitational learning theory and teaching practices that bring this theory to life and that intentionally facilitate trust, respect, and optimism in the online classroom. The theory and ideas presented in this chapter provide a foundation for online teachers in a variety of courses and disciplines to develop and adapt additional teaching activities to achieve this.

REFERENCES

Andrei, D., Oţoiu, C., Isailă, Ş., & Băban, A. (2010). What does it mean to trust your team colleague? An exploratory study using grounded theory. *Cognition, Brain, Behavior, 14*(2), 121–140.

Chant, R., Moes, R., & Ross, M. (2009). Curriculum construction and teacher empowerment: Supporting invitational education with creative problem solving. *Journal of Invitational Theory and Practice, 15*, 55–67.

Cohen, J. R. (2001). When people are the means: Negotiating with respect. *Georgetown Journal of Legal Ethics, 14*, 739–802. Retrieved from http://ssrn. com/abstract=1612756

Cook, L. (2005). Inviting teaching behaviors of clinical faculty and nursing students' anxiety. *Journal of Nursing Education, 44*(4), 156–161.

Esman, B. (2011). Mozart, and juggling dominoes. *Chemistry in Australia*, 78(3), 27–29.

Frijda, N. H. (1986). *The emotions: Studies in emotions and social interaction.* Cambridge, UK: Cambridge University Press.

Haigh, M. (2008). Coloring in the emotional language of place. *Journal of Invitational Theory and Practice*, 14, 25–40.

Haigh, M. (2011). Invitational education: Theory, research and practice. *Journal of Geography in Higher Education*, 35(2), 299–309.

Hunter, M., & Smith, K. H. (2007). Inviting school success: Invitational education and the art class. *Journal of Invitational Theory and Practice*, 13, 8–15.

Nooteboom, B. (2006). Forms, sources and processes of trust. In R. Bachmann & A. Zaheer (Eds.), *Handbook of trust research* (pp. 247–263). Northampton, MA: Edward Elgar.

Palmer-Jones, N., & Hoertdoerfer, P. (2008). Let's talk about respect. Unitarian Universalist Association Family Matters Task Force, *Taking It Home: Families and Faith* series. Retrieved from http://www.uua.org/documents/hoertdoerferpat/respect.pdf

Paxton, P. (2003). Inviting e-learning: How hard can it be? *Journal of Invitational Theory and Practice*, 9, 923–940.

Perry, B. (2006). Using photographic images as an interactive online teaching strategy. *The Internet and Higher Education*, 9(3). 229–240. doi:10.1016/j.iheduc.2006.06.008

Perry, B., & Edwards, M. (2010). Creating a culture of community in the online classroom using artistic pedagogical technologies. In G. Veletsianos (Ed.), *Emerging Technologies in Distance Education*. Edmonton: Athabasca University Press.

Purkey, W. W. (1992). An introduction to invitational theory. *Journal of Invitational Theory and Practice*, 1, 5–15.

Purkey, W. W. (2006). *Teaching class clowns (and what they can teach us)*. Thousand Oaks, CA: Corwin.

Purkey, W. W., & Novak, J. (1996). *Inviting school success: A self-concept approach to teaching, learning, and democratic practice* (3rd ed.). New York: Wadsworth.

Purkey, W. W., & Novak, J. M. (2008). *Fundamentals of invitational education*. Kennesaw, GA: International Alliance for Invitational Education.

Revere, L., & Kovach, J. V. (2011). Online technologies for engaged learning: A meaningful synthesis for educators. *Quarterly Review of Distance Education*, *12*(2), 113–124.

Riner, P. (2003). The intimate correlation of invitational education and effective classroom management. *Journal of Invitational Theory and Practice*, *9*, 41–55.

Riner, P. (2010). East or west, the goal is the same: Buddhist psychology and its potential contributions to invitational education. *Journal of Invitational Theory and Practice*, *16*, 88–104.

Schmidt, J. J. (2007). Elements of diversity in invitational practice and research. *Journal of Invitational Theory and Practice*, *13*, 16–23.

Shaw, D. E., & Siegel, B. L. (2010). Re-adjusting the kaleidoscope: The basic tenants [sic] of invitational theory and practice. *Journal of Invitational Theory and Practice*, *16*, 106–113. Retrived from http://medicine.nova.edu/~danshaw/jitp/archive/JITP_V16_2010.pdf

Stanley, P. H., Juhnke, G., & Purkey, W. W. (2004). Using an invitational theory of practice to create safe and successful schools. *Journal of Counseling and Development*, *82*(3), 302–310.

Thompson, D. R. (2004). Organizational learning in action: Becoming an inviting school. *Journal of Invitational Theory and Practice*, *10*, 52–72.

Tsukiyama, G. (1994). *The samurai's garden*. New York: St Martin's Griffin.

van Manen, M. (1990). *Researching lived experience: Human science for an action sensitive pedagogy*. London, ON: Althouse Press.

Wade, C., Cameron, B., Morgan, K., & Williams, K. (2011). Are interpersonal relationships necessary for developing trust in online group projects? *Distance Education*, *32*(3), 383–396.

Wang, C. C. (1999). Photovoice: A participatory action research strategy applied to women's health. *Journal of Women's Health*, *8*(2), 185–192.

Wang, C. C., & Burris, M. (1997). Photovoice: Concept, methodology, and use for participatory needs assessment. *Health Education Behaviour*, *24*, 369–387.

Wenger, E. (1998). *Communities of practice: Learning, meaning, and identity.* Cambridge: Cambridge University Press.

3

Constructivism: Building on What Learners Know

The word *construct* comes from the Latin prefix *com* (together) + *struere* (to pile up): to heap up together, to build or arrange. Constructivist approaches to teaching and learning are grounded in the idea that students bring valuable prior knowledge to their classes and that teachers help learners to build up that knowledge through active and personally meaningful learning activities. Teachers who embrace a constructivist approach seek ways to know students as individuals; to understand their unique ways of building, organizing, and interpreting knowledge; and to guide them toward new ways of thinking. One of the central principles of constructivism is that "individuals try to give meaning to, or construe, the perplexing maelstrom of events and ideas in which they find themselves caught up" (Candy, 1989, p. 97).

Few people are able to interpret and make sense of new professional knowledge on their own. Learning is a social process: it occurs when learners glean new insights from informed others. In online classrooms, both teachers and peers are valuable resources in this regard. Theorists such as Lev Vygotsky (1978) use the term "social constructivism" to extend the notion of individual construction of meaning, thus acknowledging input from informed others. The notion of "scaffolding" suggests that teachers and peers can offer temporary support to other individuals during their personal processes of constructing meaning.

This chapter begins with a description of social constructivism and the underlying tenets of this approach. This is followed by an explanation of some scaffolding tactics that constructivist teachers can implement to help students develop their own ways of knowing. Although learners all construct meaning differently, these strategies offer common guidelines for helping others to build knowledge.

BACKGROUND THEORY

What Is Social Constructivism?

Constructivists view knowledge as contextual and relative, and reject the notion that knowledge is an innate commodity that can be objectified or discovered. Jean Piaget, considered one of the founders of constructivism, proposed that individuals construct new knowledge in relation to past experiences (1972). Piaget believed that knowledge develops through a process of assimilating and accommodating new ideas into the schematic frameworks or ways of knowing that already exist in an individual's mind (1972).

A constructivist orientation to the nature of knowledge suggests that "knowledge is not discovered like gold or oil, but rather is constructed like cars or pyramids" (Novak & Gowan, 1984, p. 4). According to Novak (1993), constructivists "hold that knowledge is a construction based on previous knowledge and constantly evolving over time" (p. 169).

In education, a constructivist approach assumes that teaching is not a process of transmitting intact knowledge to learners. Constructivists do not view learners as empty vessels awaiting filling or blank slates awaiting words. Rather, learners are viewed as builders who are continually creating mental representations of events and experiences. This creation is learning.

Key principles of constructivist thinking that guide teaching and course design include connecting all learning activities to a larger goal, encouraging learner responsibility, and ensuring that required tasks reflect the complexities of practice (Savery & Duffy, 1996). Additionally, constructivist learning environments are expected to challenge learners' thinking. In addition to supporting what students already know, constructivist teachers lead students toward reflecting deeply, thinking in new ways, and testing their ideas against alternate views (Savery & Duffy, 1996).

Constructivist learning environments are sometimes perceived as somewhat loosely defined. Learning outcomes may not initially seem easy to measure and may not be exactly the same for each learner. However, while different learners may draw diverse conclusions and have dissimilar learning outcomes, constructivist teachers must identify and redirect any misconceptions or misinterpretations that arise during knowledge construction. In other words, teachers have an overarching responsibility for steering learners toward learning activities that might be relevant to their education.

Constructivism has been criticized for its apparent willingness to accept uncritically any and all interpretations of events. In addressing this critique, Candy (1989) emphasizes that not all constructions are equally useful or valid and that education requires people to reconstruct events and ideas in ways that lead to more functional outcomes for them. Thus, a constructivist perspective can incorporate consensually validated knowledge as well as individual knowing. This point is particularly relevant to health care professional education, where achieving a recognized standard of consensually validated knowledge is critical. There are simply some things that students in health care programs must know to be competent practitioners. For example, there is little room for creativity in taking an accurate blood pressure reading, and laboratory values have specific meaning and are not open to imaginative analysis.

While health care students must acquire certain knowledge, the process of acquiring that knowledge can be individually constructed. Given the importance of ensuring that learners are incorporating consensually validated professional knowledge, albeit in their own way and with their own subjective mental representations, it is not surprising that constructivist thinking also moves beyond the cognitive to acknowledge the profound influence that social and cultural factors can have on learning.

Understanding the "Social" in Social Constructivism

Social constructivists address the social and collaborative dimensions of learning. Building on the premise that knowledge develops in relation to past experiences, influential social constructivist theorist Lev Vygotsky (1978) emphasizes how learning is also profoundly influenced by interaction with, and help from, more knowledgeable peers. In Vygotsky's work with children, he coined the term "zone of proximal development," defining it as "the distance between the actual development level as determined by independent problem solving and the level of potential development as determined through problem solving under adult guidance or in collaboration with more capable peers" (1978, p. 86). In essence, this zone encompasses the discrepancy between what learners can achieve with social support and what they can achieve independently. Constructivist teachers can help minimize this difference through including intentional socializing experiences with informed others in course design and instruction.

Social constructivists believe that both adults and children have zones of proximal development. These zones, or ranges of ability and potential, are unique to each individual. Teachers must consider certain questions when assessing each student's particular zone of proximal development: What activities can this student do independently? What activities can this student do with assistance but not independently? And most importantly, what assistance from a teacher or peers will be most helpful in moving this student toward independence in achieving required competencies? Teachers can create this needed help through instructional scaffolding.

Instructional Scaffolding

Instructional scaffolding is a teaching strategy whereby instructors initially provide considerable support and foundational knowledge on a topic. Similar to scaffolds on construction sites, the support is temporary and is not expected to be required for long. As students need less help, demonstrate independence, and assume more responsibility for meeting their learning needs on their own, the support or scaffolding is gradually withdrawn.

In order to provide needed foundational knowledge efficiently, any instructional scaffolding must be carefully planned and must address areas that most students typically find difficult. Students need a clear understanding of the goals, purposes, and expected outcomes of learning activities. They need sequenced opportunities that expose them to new content, and they need frequent feedback on how their personal progress is being measured in relation to peers. These needs are usually met at the curricular level in health care education, but certain teaching techniques and tools can enhance the scaffolding that is structured into the online curriculum, including the personalizing of sequenced events, advance organizers, modelling, and student-led activities.

PERSONALIZING OF SEQUENCED EVENTS

Course outlines usually provide students and teachers with required content and assignments—an important part of the instructional scaffolding. However, constructivist teachers individualize curricular requirements and continually introduce relevant new disciplinary knowledge. Established teacher-initiated scaffolding approaches include modelling desired behaviours, offering explanations, inviting student participation, and verifying or clarifying student understandings (Hogan & Pressley, 1997).

In online learning environments, course guides offering choices of learning activities are particularly helpful instructional scaffolds. Legg, Adelman, Mueller, and Levitt suggest having students "decide to which of several discussion threads to respond, and allowing the student to find his or her own resources" (2009, p. 68). Although health care educators follow required curriculum and course guides, opportunities for building in creative support that personalizes these sequenced events and responds to learners' evolving needs are limitless.

ADVANCE ORGANIZERS

Constructivist teachers can create scaffolds or support for new information by emphasizing what it is about an area of content that is particularly important. Knowing aspects of a topic that can be expected to be difficult or complex, educators can organize that information in ways that offer learners a way of looking at the material in advance. Most educators create and present advance organizers such as charts, diagrams, or other visual tools for organizing and representing consensually validated knowledge into their teaching practice. A summary of course content in a concise PowerPoint or Prezi presentation is another advance organizer that incorporates a graphic or visual element.

Extending the usual teaching practice of providing general overviews or summaries of course material, theorist David Ausubel (1960, 1968) suggests that learners can come to understand ideas, concepts, and principles more deeply and more meaningfully when advance organizers include both a reminder about relevant prior knowledge and an emphasis on the relationships that exist among concepts. To this end, a learning activity that guides students to recall what they already know about a course topic is a useful advance organizer.

Mind maps and concept maps are two different kinds of graphic organizers that help learners to assimilate what they already know and what they are about to learn (Davies, 2011; Melrose, 2013). Mind maps, introduced by popular author Tony Buzan (1974), are informal intuitive diagrams used to represent a single word or idea. Mind maps, like web or spider diagrams, incorporate colours, symbols, and pictures and are often used as tools for taking notes or illustrating brainstorming activities.

By contrast, concept maps, introduced by science educators Joe Novak and Bob Gowan (1984), connect multiple words or ideas. Concept maps are hierarchical schematic diagrams that use words or symbols to represent key concepts. This tool uses linking words to show the relationship between concepts; the concept map can then be used to produce meaningful statements or propositions (Novak & Cañas, 2008). Because they illustrate the relationships, connections, and patterns among ideas, concept maps can be considered more complex advance organizers. Constructivist teachers can use advance organizers such as mind maps or concept maps both to present material to students and to evaluate how students are piecing together the new knowledge they are acquiring. When assignments invite students to synthesize what they have learned into their own advance organizers, the process of completing those assignments can encourage creativity and imagination as well as analysis.

MODELLING

Providing structures or templates that teachers themselves have found valuable, explaining concepts in relation to students' practice areas, co-writing papers, and reviewing drafts of assignments before formally grading them are all valuable instructional scaffolds that can be considered modelling. Instructional scaffolding, like any worthwhile teaching activity, requires constant attention and a willingness to relate on a personal level. In order for students to benefit fully from activities available to them, they need to know that their teachers are willing to risk modelling their own ways of approaching a task. Knowing about a teacher's in-progress projects and mistakes as well as successes can offer meaningful support and concrete examples.

Hankemeier and Van Lunen (2011) found that role-modelling can be used to promote the use of evidence-based practice with students. When teachers are willing to lead by example, they can, through demonstration, provide students with both motivation and specific knowledge acquired. The model provided by the educator becomes a structure upon which learners can construct their own way of proceeding in various real-life situations.

STUDENT-LED ACTIVITIES

Online classrooms can provide ideal opportunities for students to assume leadership roles with the class group. Although verbal and nonverbal contextual cues may not be as clear in online asynchronous text-based discussions or even when using synchronous technology such as conference calls (Karpova, Correia, & Baran, 2009), student-led activities in online classrooms can help generate innovative ideas and active involvement (Baran & Correia, 2009). However, the timing of these activities is critical. In the first few weeks of the course, it is critical that teachers model the kind of facilitation approaches that they expect from the students and intentionally prepare students for their leadership role. And, as Baran and Correia (2009) emphasize, perhaps the most important role of teachers is to be active participants in the student-led activities.

Summary

As noted above, constructivist approaches to teaching and learning, and social constructivism in particular, assume that knowledge is constructed. Learners bring valuable existing knowledge to their learning experiences, and teachers are expected to build on that knowledge by providing personally meaningful activities. Knowing that learning can be profoundly influenced by informed others such as teachers and peers, constructivist educators plan for and facilitate opportunities for helpful social interaction. Throughout the learning process, instructional scaffolding, or temporary supports, are available. These scaffolds initially provide substantive foundational knowledge, offer sequenced opportunities for understanding new ideas, and are gradually withdrawn as learners construct their own ways of understanding the material. Learning activities are designed to link to students' personal goals, connect theory to practice, and invite deep and critical reflection.

Constructivist learning environments incorporate consensually validated knowledge and professional practice standards, and competencies are comprehensively evaluated. Students' misconceptions are identified and redirected. Learners are viewed as having a unique and individual zone of ability where they are able to complete an activity independently. Working collaboratively, students and teachers determine what assistance is needed to move toward increasing that zone of independence. Instructional scaffolding methods that support a learner's growing independence include the personalizing of sequenced events structured into the curriculum and course outline, advance organizers such as mind maps and concept maps, modelling and sharing in-progress projects, and student-led activities.

TEACHING ACTIVITIES AND STRATEGIES CONGRUENT WITH CONSTRUCTIVIST THEORY

The following discussion expands on scaffolding tactics that constructivist teachers can readily implement in their online classes. These techniques are grounded in social constructivist thinking, involve learners in active and creative ways, and are geared toward promoting learner independence.

Creating Instructional Scaffolds

ADVANCE ORGANIZERS: MIND MAPS AND CONCEPT MAPS

Mind maps and concept maps are advance organizers that provide the kind of scaffolding or support that can assist learners in moving toward completing an activity successfully and independently. When we teach students about mind and concept maps, showing them a sketch of our thinking—a visual representation of the relationships among ideas—can be much more effective than simply explaining them verbally. Creating a mind map begins with identifying a central word or concept and then using a branching structure to expand on the concept, as illustrated in the mind map of social constructivism shown in figure 2. Colours and pictures can be included. Online tools with mapping templates are readily available for students and teachers. However, learners particularly value their teacher's more informal visuals.

Mind maps and concept maps are different. Buzan and Buzan (2006) developed mind maps as an informal means of exploring a specific idea by brainstorming key points associated with that idea. In contrast, the concept maps of Novak and Gowan (1984), sometimes referred to as Novakian concept maps, were developed to illustrate several key concepts and the relationships among these concepts, which are specified by the use of carefully chosen linking words.

Constructivism

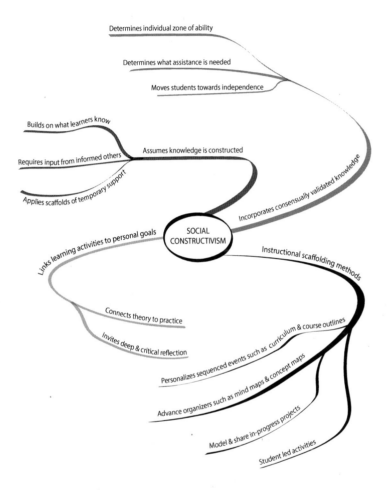

Determines individual zone of ability

Determines what assistance is needed

Moves students towards independence

Builds on what learners know

Requires input from informed others

Assumes knowledge is constructed

Applies scaffolds of temporary support

Incorporates consensually validated knowledge

Links learning activities to personal goals

SOCIAL CONSTRUCTIVISM

Instructional scaffolding methods

Connects theory to practice

Invites deep & critical reflection

Personalizes sequenced events such as curriculum & course outlines

Advance organizers such as mind maps & concept maps

Model & share in-progress projects

Student led activities

Figure 2. Mind map of social constructivism.

Figure 3 is a concept map that Michael Zeilik, of the Department of Physics and Astronomy at the University of New Mexico, created to explain concept maps. The concepts identified in Zeilik's map are linked in such a way that following the arrows produces a continuous statement, such as "Concept maps can be used for classroom assessment by revealing the knowledge structure of students . . ." Without the appropriate explanatory linking words, Novakian concept maps are incomplete.

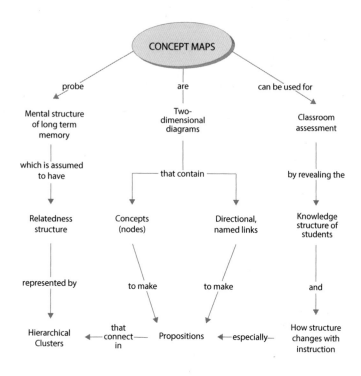

Figure 3. Concept map of concept maps. Source: Zeilik (n.d.). Reproduced with permission.

CROSSWORD PUZZLES

Crossword puzzles are excellent scaffolding tools for concrete or instrumental knowledge construction. With a sense of simplicity and playfulness, they require learners to apply vocabulary, recall definitions, differentiate among similar terms, and spell correctly. According to blogger Kerry Jones, visual learners feel satisfied after completing puzzles, auditory learners enjoy the step-by-step reasoning, and kinesthetic learners appreciate the required multitasking (Jones, 2007). Crossword puzzles offer online health care learners opportunities to integrate the vocabulary of their discipline.

Both ready-made puzzles and programs designed to create online puzzles are widely available. An Internet search with the term "make a crossword puzzle" yields several free programs suitable for educators at all levels. Most programs require simply typing in a word and a definition. Similarly, an Internet search with the term "crossword puzzle nursing" (substitute any health care discipline) yields a selection of ready-made puzzles.

MODELLING AN IN-PROGRESS PROJECT

Students appreciate knowing how their teachers construct meaning. Modelling in the online classroom can include activities as simple as discussing how work is progressing on a project in which the instructor is involved. In text-based discussion forums, a teacher's experience of writing reports or papers can be shared, or a description of current work can be provided, with comments on both what is going well and what is not going well. Students usually appreciate instructors taking the risk of sharing what they have found especially difficult. Did they feel conflicted or puzzled? How did they overcome challenges and barriers? Which strategies worked better than others? It is important to note that the goal of instructional modelling is to provide personal and real examples that learners can relate to and possibly emulate. Thoughtful examples that are clearly relevant to course content currently under discussion are most useful as constructivist teaching tools.

From the Field: Modelling Through Being Visible

Carol Anderson focuses on modelling for students through ongoing purposeful communication—specifically, weekly unit introductions and summaries. This process demonstrates skills such as scholarly writing, referencing, thematic analysis, and organization. In addition to modelling, it shows students that she is actively participating in the course and is available to them. In a face-to-face setting, it would be called "being visible."

Each week, Carol writes an introduction to that week's unit reiterating the objectives of the module. She refers to the previous week (or weeks) in an effort to link the modules and show how they build on each other. Sometimes, Carol uses personal experiences relevant to the topic, both to inform students and to help them get to know her. In this way, she models appropriate social interaction and personal disclosure in online learning environments. In the weekly introduction, which provides a starting point to the week's discussion, Carol often comments on the progress of assignments, reminds students of due dates, and offers help with any questions the students may have.

In a posting to the class at the end of each week, Carol summarizes some of the points that are most directly related to the objectives for the unit. In each of these summaries, she recognizes at least three students for their comments on a specific item. In so doing, she models the importance of recognizing the contributions of others in building a healthy learning environment. To facilitate this recognition, she keeps a private log of the students she mentions each week so that she has recognized everyone in the class individually by the end of the course. Carol sometimes adds questions or suggestions for deeper reflection or discussion to her end-of-the-week summary, role-modelling the importance of continued learning and building on existing knowledge.

Carol has received many positive comments from students on this teaching technique. One student said, "The instructor sharing some end of the week reflections demonstrated an interest and level of participation that was appreciated." Another student noticed that Carol was role-modelling, commenting, "Carol modelled many of the strategies and concepts we discussed. Additionally, the instructor challenged the class to achieve!" Finally, a student in the course wrote, "Carol's introductions and summaries launched things nicely and brought them back to earth again."

Facilitating Students' Creation of Instructional Scaffolds

STUDENT-LED SEMINARS

As emphasized earlier, student-led seminars or activities are more likely to be successful if teachers model the kind of facilitation they expect, prepare learners for leadership, and actively participate in the student-led seminars. Most online courses have a discussion component that could be facilitated by students. It is important that all students have equal opportunities to participate in the roles of both leader and follower in course seminars. Working in pairs or small groups of three or four is optimal for leading a class of 15 to 30 in discussion. One straightforward, universal, and efficient way to prepare any group of students for leading seminars is to present Savery and Duffy's (1996) eight principles of instructional design. Table 1, which can be used as a handout, summarizes these principles. Students can be encouraged to plan, implement, and evaluate their seminar in relation to these principles, with the instructor checking in frequently and maintaining an ongoing dialogue with the student leaders as they are preparing for their seminar. Formative evaluation at the completion of the student-led seminar can be an important element in making this activity a learning experience.

Table 1. Principles of instructional design

---

1. *Anchor all activities to a larger task or problem.*

   The purpose of the activity and how it links to "real world" issues must be clear to learners.

2. *Support the learner in developing ownership for the overall problem or task.*

   Either solicit problems from learners to use as stimuli for learning activities or present a problem in a way that learners will readily adopt as their own.

3. *Design an authentic task.*

   An authentic task is one in which the cognitive demands are consistent with the demands of the environment for which we are preparing the learner.

4. *Design the task and the learning environment to reflect the complexity of the environment in which learners will be required to function when they have finished their program.*

   Rather than simplify the environment for the learner, support the complexities they will face.

5. *Give the learner ownership of the process used to develop a solution.*

   Rather than dictating a procedure or method to use, challenge the learner's thinking about how to solve a problem.

6. *Design the learning environment to support and challenge the learner's thinking.*

   Just as a coach or consultant might, support how learners are going about their problem-solving efforts and question their rationale.

7. *Encourage the testing of ideas against alternative views and contexts.*

   Given that knowledge is socially negotiated, ensure that alternative views are available.

8. *Provide opportunity for and support reflection on both the content learned and the learning process.*

   Keeping in mind that the goal of instruction is to develop independent learners by creating opportunities to reflect on the process of learning, or "how" learning occurred, as well as on the content, or "what" was learned.

SOURCE: Adapted from Savery and Duffy (1996).

SOCRATIC SEMINARS

One popular student-led activity involves learners presenting content relevant to a specific topic and then posing questions for their classmates to discuss. Socratic seminars extend this idea by paying particular attention to the types of questions that are posed. Students may need some assistance with creating questions that fit the Socratic method of teaching. Socratic questions challenge individuals to think deeply and critically about concepts often taken for granted.

A Socratic dialogue is fitting when student presentations to their peers involve difficult issues or ethical or moral dilemmas. Questions in Socratic seminars are expected to challenge participants to make comparisons, give evidence for cause-and-effect relationships, and provide suggestions for why an issue or practice might be realistic or unrealistic. While "right answers" are not expected, participants must demonstrate that they are integrating content from the presentation and from their own investigations into their responses. Socratic questions draw out the beliefs of participants and challenge students to consider ideas from more than one point of view. To guide students toward crafting authentic Socratic questions for their peers to discuss, the following summary of Paul's taxonomy of Socratic question types can be provided as a handout.

Table 2. Taxonomy of Socratic question types

1. *Seeking clarification.*

   Questions that aim to elicit additional information on concepts:

   As an individual or as a professional group, how do we usually define or explain _____? What do we already know about _____?

2. *Probing assumptions.*

   Questions that expose the presuppositions or unquestioned beliefs that ground thinking:

   How can we verify or disprove that assumption? How did that assumption come to be part of our practice? What would happen if _____?

3. *Probing rationale, reasons, and evidence.*

   Questions that dig into rationale for arguments and uncover assumptions:

   What is the reason we do _____? Would this practice stand up in court? How might it be refuted?

4. *Questioning viewpoints and perspectives.*

   Questions that invite consideration of other equally valid points of view:

   Another way of looking at this is _____: does this seem reasonable? Who benefits most from _____? What effect would _____ have?

5. *Probing implications and consequences.*
   Questions that challenge the desirability of an argument's logical implications:

   What are the consequences of _____? How do we find out _____? Can we generalize from _____ to _____?

6. *Asking questions about the question.*
   Questions that reflect and extend the initial questions:

   What other questions about _____ should we be asking?

SOURCE: Adapted from Paul (1995) and Paul and Elder (2006).

LUNCH WITH THE THEORISTS

Student-led activities online can also include role play. Melrose (2006) designed an activity inviting learners to imagine that they have an opportunity to have lunch with three theorists. As a way of presenting theoretical concepts to one another, students join a selected theorist for a virtual lunch. They begin by visualizing what it might be like to sit across the table from a theorist whose work is widely read. They consider how the theorist might explain his or her views in an informal way, what real-life guidance on immediate practice issues the theorist might offer, and instances in which this theorist's ideas would probably not be helpful. At the conclusion of the virtual lunch, the student shares the perspectives gained with the class in a discussion forum beginning with the words "Today I had lunch with _____." In student-led seminars, student presenters can be encouraged to tap into affective learning domains, to use humour whenever possible, and to have fun.

As variations on this activity, each student presenter in the seminar could assume the role of a theorist, offer comments on a practice issue, and respond to questions that the class group might have. Alternatively, the seminar group could present a vignette of a group of theorists conversing over lunch. With the goal of bringing a theory to life by coming to know the person behind the theory, the presentation could be shared simply as a script. More complex presentations could be developed by acting out the roles in podcasts or videos. However, the essence of the "Lunch with the Theorists" activity is to "conceptualize well-known theorists in a familiar everyday activity and de-mystify the ideas these individuals espouse" (Melrose, 2006, p. 1). Rather than simply reiterating published explanations of a theory, this activity both personalizes the people who created the theories and reveals the immediate relevance of their ideas to current practice.

TWITTER JOURNAL CLUB

Many health care professionals are familiar with journal clubs, where a group of individuals meet face to face to exchange insights in relation to scholarly journal articles. For this activity, all members of a student group could read a particular article and then present a group summary, or individuals could each summarize a different article to help inform the group. Presentations are brief and discussion about relevance and application to practice usually follows. In clinical settings, journal clubs can help inform practitioners about current research and new ways of thinking.

In online student-led seminars, the journal club activity can be adapted to Twitter. (Twitter accounts can be created free of charge at twitter.com.) Student leaders can transfer the traditional face-to-face journal club process to an online group by distributing to classmates a brief presentation of an article and then leading a practice-related discussion using Twitter. Confining summarized journal article comments to the 140-characters maximum allowed in a tweet requires participants to sift through large volumes of information and identify priority ideas. Similarly, limiting practice-related discussion comments in this way requires succinct and precise expression of priority points.

Student leaders can be asked to establish clear directions for their online Twitter journal club. For example, a group might decide to provide the class with a link to a journal article as well as three tweets, each one summarizing a different idea emphasized in the publication. The group could then require each member of the class to respond with at least two tweets to one of the ideas, with each tweet linking the point from the article to practice and describing how the point was useful or not useful. The Twitter discussion of the selected article would be asynchronous and ongoing, but confined to a specified time period, perhaps five days.

The activity of using Twitter to discuss journal articles can be implemented in a variety of creative ways. However, as a constructivist learning activity, it must go beyond simply presenting an article and then receiving tweets from peers. Student leaders can be instructed on how to provide scaffolding by organizing the tweets into groups or general categories. As a way of closing the activity, the student and/ or the instructor can identify common themes. Perhaps the majority of the class did not feel that the ideas in an article were relevant for practice. Did any of the tweets seem to influence the direction the discussion? Was there a group of tweets that opened new areas of inquiry? And finally, in the interest of inclusiveness, alternate opportunities can be created for members of the group who choose not to use Twitter so that they too can contribute their 140-character messages to the discussions.

USE A MERLOT RESOURCE IN A STUDENT-LED ACTIVITY

The Multimedia Educational Resource for Learning and Online Teaching (MERLOT) website (www.merlot.org) offers health care professionals a useful collection of free, peer-reviewed teaching and learning resources. Student leaders can use MERLOT to devise a sharing activity for seminars they are expected to lead. They might ask their classmates to browse through the health sciences section of the website and post one resource that could be implemented in their practice. The activity could also include requiring participants to respond to at least one classmate's posted resource. Students can be reminded of the importance of incorporating analytic discussion in both the posted resources and the responses.

CONCLUSION

As we have seen, constructivist thinking is a process in which learners build on what they already know by participating in active and personally relevant learning experiences. As theorist Jean Piaget (1972) asserts, constructivism is based on the notion that knowledge develops when new ideas are assimilated into the schematic frameworks or ways of knowing that already exist. Although a constructivist perspective highlights personal construction of meaning, in health care education, the approach must also incorporate consensually validated knowledge, and teachers are expected to identify and redirect any misconceptions on the part of the students.

Social constructivism acknowledges the profound impact that informed others, such as teachers and peers, can have on meaningful learning. By creating opportunities for students to engage in helpful interactions with peers, teachers offer possibilities for looking at the world in new and different ways. Theorist Lev Vygotsky (1978) believed that learners have a unique and individual zone of ability (or "zone of proximal development"). Within this zone, a learner is able to complete some activities independently but requires social support for others. As constructivist teachers seek to increase learners' zones of independence, they invite members of the class to interact and exchange insights with one another.

Instructional scaffolding, or offering temporary support until learners are able to complete activities independently, is needed most in areas that students typically find difficult. At the curricular level, scaffolds provide foundational disciplinary knowledge through sequenced events such as required assignments identified on course outlines. At the instructional level, scaffolds include personalizing those sequenced events and linking them to students' individual goals. Instructional scaffolding tactics that teachers can readily implement in their online classrooms include creating advance organizers, making crossword puzzles, modelling, and establishing student-led activities. Advance organizers, such as simple mind maps that illustrate one key idea or more complex concept maps that illustrate relationships among concepts, can be used to organize consensually validated knowledge. Teachers can help students to make connections between theory and practice by modelling processes that they have found valuable, sharing their in-progress projects, and describing their mistakes. The scaffolding approach that is perhaps the most likely to generate deep and critical reflection is requiring students themselves to lead class activities. Four examples of student-led activities are leading Socratic seminars, having lunch with the theorists, organizing a Twitter journal club, and sharing a MERLOT resource. Constructivist approaches to teaching and learning call upon teachers to know their students. By looking at the world through students' eyes, educators can creatively, collaboratively, and even playfully support their ways of knowing and growing.

REFERENCES

Ausubel, D. P. (1960). The use of advance organizers in the learning and retention of meaningful verbal material. *Journal of Educational Psychology*, *51*, 267–272.

Ausubel, D. P. (1968). *Educational psychology: A cognitive view*. New York: Holt, Rinehart, & Winston.

Baran, E., & Correia, A.-P. (2009). Student-led facilitation strategies in online discussion. *Distance Education*, *30*(3), 339–361.

Buzan, T. (1974). *Use your head.* London: BBC Books.

Buzan, T., & Buzan, B. (2006). *The mind map book.* Boston: Pearson Education.

Candy, P. (1989). Constructivism and the study of self-direction in adult learning. *Studies in the Education of Adults, 21,* 95–116.

Davies, M. (2011). Concept mapping, mind mapping, and argument mapping: What are the differences and why do they matter? *Higher Education, 62*(3), 279–301.

Hankemeier, D., & Van Lunen, B. (2011). Approved clinical instructors' perspectives on implementation strategies in evidence-based practice for athletic training students. *Journal of Athletic Training, 46*(6), 655–664.

Hogan, K., & Pressley, M. (Eds.). (1997). *Scaffolding student learning: Instructional approaches and issues.* Cambridge, MA: Brookline Books.

Jones, K. (2007, September 10). *Teaching with Crossword Puzzles* [blog]. Retrieved from http://vocabulary.co.il/blog/learning_vocabulary/teaching-with-crossword-puzzles/

Karpova, E., Correia, A.-P., & Baran, E. (2009). Learn to use and use to learn: Technology in virtual collaboration experience. *The Internet and Higher Education, 12*(1), 45–52.

Legg, T. J., Adelman, D., Mueller, D., & Levitt, C. (2009). Constructivist strategies in online distance education in nursing. *Journal of Nursing Education, 48*(2), 64–69.

Melrose, S. (2006). Lunch with the theorists: A clinical learning activity. *Nurse Educator, 31*(4), 147–148.

Melrose, S. (2013). Facilitating constructivist learning environments using mind maps and concept maps as advance organizers. *JPACTe: Journal for the Practical Application of Constructivist Theory in Education, 7*(1). Retrieved from http://www.jpacte.org/uploads/9/0/0/6/9006355/2013-1-melrose.pdf

Novak, J. D. (1993). Human constructivism: A unification of psychological and epistemological phenomena in meaning making. *International Journal of Personal Construct Psychology, 6,* 167–193.

Novak, J. D., & Cañas, A. J. (2008). *The theory underlying concept maps and how to construct and use them.* Technical Report IHMC CmapTools 2006-

01 Rev 01-2008. Florida: Institute for Human and Machine Cognition. Retrieved from http://cmap.ihmc.us/Publications/ResearchPapers/ TheoryUnderlyingConceptMaps.pdf

Novak, J. D., & Gowan, B. (1984). *Learning how to learn*. Cambridge, UK: Cambridge University Press.

Paul, R. (1995). *Critical thinking: How to prepare students for a rapidly changing world*. Santa Rosa, CA: Foundation for Critical Thinking.

Paul, R., & Elder, L. (2006). *The thinker's guide to the art of Socratic questioning*. Santa Rosa, CA: Foundation for Critical Thinking. Retrieved from http:// www.criticalthinking.org/TGS_files/SocraticQuestioning2006.pdf

Piaget, J. (1972). *Psychology and epistemology: Toward a theory of knowledge*. Harmondsworth, UK: Penguin.

Savery, J., & Duffy, T. (1996). Problem-based learning: An instructional method and its constructivist framework. In B. Wilson (Ed.), *Constructivist learning environments: Case studies in instructional design* (pp. 135–148). Englewood Cliffs, NJ: Educational Technology.

Vygotsky, L. S. (1978). *Mind and society: The development of higher psychological processes*. Cambridge, MA: Harvard University Press.

Zeilik, M. (n.d.). Concept mapping. Retrieved from http://www.flaguide.org/ extra/download/cat/conmap/conmap.pdf.

4

Connectivism: Learning by Forming Connections

Learning is not limited to formal environments in which educators provide students with information. Connectivist thinking invites us to imagine possibilities for self-directed learners to use Web 2.0 technology to create informal networks. Grounded in the notion that, in this digital age, knowledge is available all around us, connectivism holds that learners will connect with information, activities, and individuals through technological processes that they find interesting and efficient. These connections often result in incidental and unexpected learning that complements the learning associated with traditional modes of instruction.

Connectivism has been described as a theory that "emphasizes the importance of non-human appliances, hardware and software, and network connections for human learning. The theory stresses the development of 'metaskills' for evaluating and managing information and network connections, and notes the importance of information pattern recognition as a learning strategy" (Couros, 2009, p. 233). As health care teachers, we know that our students must make sense of vast quantities of rapidly changing information. Connectivism, with its emphasis on knowing how to use technology to find needed information, to network, and to judge the relevance of information, is tailor-made for us. George Siemens, the founder of connectivism, could well have had the education of health professionals in mind when he wrote:

> Learning occurs as a result of reflection on, and validation of, content ... this process is most often initiated through interaction. In this model (and online), content is not less important. The difference is in how content is explored ... and to a degree who provides it—teacher, student, or both. Effective teaching requires equipping students with the skills and beliefs to be able to provide for their own learning. (Siemens, 2002; ellipses in original)

This focus on learning as a process of interaction was the beginning of the theory of connectivism.

In December 2004, Siemens posted his first article on this new learning theory, "Connectivism: A Learning Theory for the Digital Age." In this concept paper, Siemens explains the underpinnings of connectivism: "Including technology and connection making as learning activities begins to move learning theories into a digital age. We can no longer personally experience and acquire [the] learning that we need to act. We derive our competence from forming connections" (2004, "An Alternative Theory," para. 1). In other words, much of what we need to know now exists in virtual form, beyond the reach of direct experience. Then, drawing on chaos theory (Gleick, 1987), self-organization theory (Rocha, 1998), and Barabási's (2002) network theory (order is created by patterning and organizing information, a process in which certain pieces of information are assigned a higher value than others), Siemens further refined the theory of connectivism. To promote discussion of the emerging theory within the broader education community, in 2005 he established a website (www.connectivism.ca) devoted to the exploration of connectivism. In "Learning in Synch with Life" (2006), Siemens examined challenges currently faced by educators and found them similar to those experienced by organizations. For example, today's learners and educators are experiencing evolving societal pressures, immersion in constantly changing technology, rapid information growth requiring the effective use of technology and networks to store information, the globalization of interactions, and the breakdown of centralization in order to allow for adaptation and growth. Siemens concluded that these pressures demand an examination of how we teach and learn in the twenty-first century.

BACKGROUND THEORY

What Is Connectivism?

Siemens identified eight fundamental principles of connectivism:

- Learning and knowledge rests [sic] in a diversity of opinions.

- Learning is a process of connecting specialized nodes or information sources.

- Learning may reside in non-human appliances.

- [The] capacity to know more is more critical than what is currently known.

- Nurturing and maintaining connections is needed to facilitate continual learning.

- [The] ability to see connections between fields, ideas, and concepts is a core skill.

- Currency (accurate, up-to-date knowledge) is the intent of all connectivist learning activities.

- Decision-making is a learning process. Choosing what to learn and the meaning of incoming information is seen through the lens of a shifting reality. While there is a right answer now, it may be wrong tomorrow due to alterations in the information climate affecting the decision. (2004, "Connectivism," para. 3)

In the same paper, Siemens introduced the idea of networked learning, that is, learning as a process of network creation. A network consists of two basic elements: nodes and connections. Siemens defined a node as "any element that can be connected to any other element" and a connection as "any type of link between nodes" (2005, p. 5). As he explains, "Virtually any element that we can scrutinize or experience can become node. Thoughts, feelings, interactions with others, and new data and information can be seen as nodes. The aggregation of these nodes results in a network" (2005, p. 6). More specifically, he described networks as having the following characteristics or elements:

- Content (data or information)

- Interaction (tentative connection forming)

- Static nodes (stable knowledge structure)

- Dynamic nodes (continually changing based on new information and data)

- Self-updating nodes (nodes which are tightly linked to their original information source, resulting in a high level of currency, i.e., up to date)

- Emotive elements (emotions that influence the prospect of connection and hub formations). (2005, p. 7)

According to Siemens, the connections within a network are strengthened by emotion, motivation, exposure, patterning, logic, and experience. All of these nodes and connections are influenced by socialization and technology.

According to the theory of connectivism, learning is an activity that consists in forging connections and thus creating networks. Learning is ubiquitous, and it takes place continuously. It may result from deliberate action on the part of an individual, or it may occur in random or haphazard ways. However, as we saw, connectivism acknowledges "the importance of information pattern recognition as a learning strategy" (Couros 2009, p. 233). This pattern recognition can be actualized at the individual or group level; when the process occurs at the group level, the group becomes a networked community. As Stephen Downes puts it, "Knowledge is a network phenomenon. To 'know' something is to be organized in a certain way, to exhibit patterns of connectivity. To 'learn' is to acquire certain patterns. This is as true for a community as it is for an individual" (2006, "The Semantic Condition," para. 1).

Stephen Downes entered the connectivist discussion in a 2005 blog post, in which he argues that, in addition to qualitative and quantitative knowledge, we must include a third type in the domain of knowledge, which he called distributed, or connective, knowledge:

> Distributed knowledge adds a third major category to this domain, knowledge that could be described as connective. A property of one entity must lead to or become a property of another entity in order for them to be considered connected; the knowledge that results from such connections is connective knowledge. (2005, sec. a, para. 2)

Furthermore, Downes stresses, "Connective knowledge requires an interaction. More to the point, connective knowledge is knowledge *of* the connection" (2005, sec. a, para. 6).

Distributive knowledge, or distributive cognition, is not new to the educational psychology literature. In 1998, the concept was reviewed by Hewett and Scardamalia, who discuss schooling as "communities grounded in the practice of knowledge building" (p. 75). In that early Internet era, these authors, citing Pea (1993), indicate an evolution over time in technology supporting distributed learning: "Textbooks, notebooks, rulers, the organization of desks, and the writing on blackboards and bulletin boards are seen as cultural artifacts that carry intelligence in them" (Pea, as cited in Hewett and Scardamalia, 1998, p. 76).

In sum, the theory of connectivism as articulated by Siemens has at least some foundation in the idea of distributed knowledge. Connectivism is a theory of learning that is about more than the individual and more than content. This theory speaks to learning as a result of connections formed among ideas, people, and experiences, connections that the learner has been able to sort and pattern into meaning.

How Is Connectivism Experienced in Online Learning?

Online learners start alone and create links among nodes of information and people as they seek to understand concepts or phenomena. A new skill set in online learning requires learners to find information and to figure out if and how the new knowledge fits into the networks they are developing. Connectivism stresses two important skills that contribute to learning: the ability to seek out current information and the ability to filter secondary and extraneous information (Siemens, 2008).

In the digital arena, the amount of information and the number of networks of people are virtually limitless. As the connective experience progresses, learners filter new information as it relates to patterns forming in their minds about topics relevant to their courses and learning needs. Students use the filters of their own values, beliefs, and perspectives to contextualize newly discovered information. Each connectivist learner develops an individual knowledge base focused on his or her own learning goals. Knowing that this type of learning may, at least in part, be informal learning that does not take place within the designated course structure, connectivist teachers need to tune in to their students' unique motivations and interests. Connectivist thinking suggests that achieving a robust individual knowledge base related to a subject is powered by learners themselves and requires motivation and effort on the part of students.

Assessment of connectivist learning is challenging when criteria traditionally used to assess and value learning are applied to judge whether a student has achieved an effective learning network. In health care education, students must be able not only to articulate what they know but also to provide relevant evidence from credible sources in order to support their professional decisions and actions. Information derived from RSS feeds, Twitter, Facebook, blogs, MySpace postings, videos, and other Web 2.0 tools may or may not be accurate. In health care, misinformation could be life-threatening. Thus, if connectivist approaches to learning are to be valuable, the information gathered must be reliable. Learners may need help from their instructors in the form of feedback, guidance, role-modelling, and moral support to become competent in locating appropriate sources of information and then evaluating that information. Additionally, although learners may recognize their own tremendous growth and learning, it will not always be transparent to external evaluators. Furthermore, as Siemens concludes, "the capacity to know is more critical than what is actually known" (2008, para. 6), and this is something for which traditional education has not developed assessment criteria. When they begin to think as connectivists, students and educators may need to undergo a paradigm shift in their beliefs about how online learning occurs and how it is measured.

According to Siemens, then, connectivist online learning occurs within a distributed technological network that includes a focus on social interaction among participants. Learning is a dynamic and ongoing process that involves recognizing and interpreting patterns. Learners gain knowledge by remixing the content of their existing networks and then adding to their knowledge base by making new connections between what they know and what they discover. Knowledge transfer occurs by connecting to (adding) nodes and making informed judgements about what is relevant and accurate. Connectivist learning theory is well suited to learning about complex subjects in a field where knowledge is rapidly changing and where diverse and abundant knowledge sources are available. Learners in health care disciplines must develop ways of using technology to find credible information and to filter that information efficiently and effectively in order to make connections—that is, in order to learn.

TEACHING ACTIVITIES AND STRATEGIES CONGRUENT WITH CONNECTIVISM

The following teaching practices are grounded in connectivist theory and can facilitate health care professionals' learning. Since technology and networks are both essential components of connectivism, these activities and techniques are presented under those two categories.

Using Technology Creatively to Connect

SEE ONE, DO ONE, TEACH ONE—WITH TECHNOLOGY

Given the centrality of technology in connectivist thinking, the well-known health care teaching strategy of "see one, do one, teach one" can help keep online learning environments current. The strategy involves observing an action ("see one"), implementing the action ("do one"), and then showing a colleague how to implement the action ("teach one").

New ways of establishing digital connections emerge daily, making it difficult for institutions to keep up. Currently, digital connections are made through Internet forums, weblogs, social blogs, micro-blogging, wikis, social networks, podcasts, virtual game worlds, virtual social worlds, and social media websites. This list changes constantly as new technologies for connecting emerge. Rather than relying on educational program infrastructure to stay current, instructors can create a short activity requiring students to observe how a technological application works (see one). Then, the students practice working with it (do one), and ultimately, they demonstrate it to the class or someone they know (teach one). The emphasis is kept on the possibilities that the application offers for communication and connection among learners. The students can also be asked to evaluate the technological application in relation to their practice. The activity concludes with an online discussion question such as "Is this application accessible, relevant, and worthwhile in furthering your professional knowledge and/or networks?"

WEB QUEST OR DISCOVERIES FORUM

An online forum titled "Web Quest" or "Discoveries" can be used to encourage online students to investigate available information on a topic and make connections between the new information and what they already know. The students search online resources to find scholarly sources that they believe relate to a course topic. Based on their discoveries, they contribute links to published peer-reviewed papers, credible videos and podcasts, or other resources to the forum. Students provide a short written description with their contribution of how they used technology to make their "discovery" and to describe the connection they see between the content of their submission and what they already know about the topic. Other students may use the contributions to the forum in their own learning.

WORKING WITH WIKIS

A wiki is a tool that invites multiple users into a single online space or document. Each individual who has access can edit or add to the web page or document, facilitating collaboration. Wikis can, for example, be used to accumulate information that will be available to an entire group, with students adding items or resources to a list or chart. A wiki is also an excellent tool for scheduling group activities: each participant can indicate the times at which he or she is available. In addition to such relatively simple uses, students can use wikis to peer review scholarly work (Park et al. 2010) or to participate in a group assignment. A quick explanation of wikis and how to use them can be found in the YouTube video "Wikis in Plain English" (http://www.youtube.com/watch?v=-dnLooTdmLY).

JOIN A MOOC

The massive open online course (MOOC), a relatively new teaching and learning technology, has received a great deal of press recently. The original MOOCs, facilitated by George Siemens, Stephen Downes, and David Cormier, were semi-structured events around the theme of education and were open to anyone and everyone who found the website and logged on. Participants found themselves on a wiki page with multiple links branching off to specific interest areas. Within interest areas, individual participants created blogs, Facebook pages, and Twitter streams to collaborate and share ideas and to network. The content was created and refined during the process.

Recently, MOOCs have been embraced by professors, consortiums, and private vendors as a way to transmit content to a large number of people simultaneously. A system of badges or assignments is embedded in some of the MOOCs to enable the granting of credit for completion of specific objectives. Although this type of MOOC still offers potential for a variety of student interaction, it defines content and process more clearly and therefore real knowledge creation is less likely.

Forming Relevant Networks

IN-DEPTH INTRODUCTIONS: WHAT IS YOUR FAVOURITE _____?

Since social interaction is crucial to connectivist learning, teaching strategies that encourage class participants to get to know one another are foundational. Interventions that allow geographically distributed learners and teachers to share details about their professional backgrounds and personal interests and aptitudes are precursors to students engaging with one another socially within the online course. One teaching approach that may facilitate this is encouraging in-depth introductions. As we emphasize throughout this book, introductions are critically important and can take various forms. For example, from a connectivist theoretical perspective, students may be invited to share one or more photos of themselves involved in an activity they enjoy. The photos may include family members, friends, pets, or images of their homes. Students could be asked to share a photo of a favourite item (for example, a T-shirt, teapot, painting, car, location, or flower) and explain why it is special to them. Students may also share the titles of songs they currently enjoy or the name of a book or movie they have read or seen more than once. This sharing usually reveals details about students that may not be apparent in a short introduction, thus providing more nodes for connection. When class participants know one another on a more personal level, existing connections will become apparent and interactions may follow. In addition, instructors can convey their membership in the group by introducing themselves in a creative way and sharing appropriate details about their values, interests, and priorities.

PROFILES THAT POP

Social media sites such as Facebook, LinkedIn, Twitter, Bebo, and MySpace allow users to create profiles that illustrate who they are, including their interests and perhaps even others who are part of their network. Knowing the importance of both technology and networking within connectivist thinking, instructors can invite students to post "profiles that pop" on these sites. Younger learners, those in paraprofessional programs, or students just beginning the process of socializing into their chosen heath care field may have more experience with creating personal profiles using social media than with creating professional profiles. However, the informal and tacit knowledge that learners all have about the kind of online presence they want to convey is invaluable. A well-crafted profile, one that "pops," can encourage connections from interested others. In most health care disciplines, establishing boundaries between personal and professional profiles is an important topic of discussion. After they have drafted their profiles, learners can share their drafts with others in the group and exchange feedback about the kinds of impressions the profiles make.

ONLINE TRADING CARDS

Youth are often familiar with "trading cards" that portray sports personalities and athletic heroes. A trading card may have a picture of a baseball or hockey player, a short history of the featured player, and the player's sport statistics in terms of touchdowns, goals scored, and so on. The object of actually trading the cards with others is to acquire the most prized or popular cards as part of one's card collection. This activity can be adapted to the online learning environment as an ice-breaking activity among students and between students and the instructor.

In this activity, students are invited to create their own personal trading cards by logging on to the Big Huge Labs trading card web page at http://bighugelabs.com/deck.php. The name of their trading card is their own name. Each student uploads a picture to share with fellow students and the instructor. In the description area of the card, students provide information about themselves (such as interests, hobbies, or pets) and the place where they would like to work after graduating. The students then save their trading card to their own computer and upload it to an online discussion forum within the course that is solely for the trading card activity. Each student creates his or her own thread. All class members are then invited to respond to the trading cards of at least two other students. Instructors can also engage in this activity to help students to get to know them better.

PERSONAL PORTFOLIO DEVELOPMENT

From the connectivist point of view, learners create their learning (or connections) to fulfill their unique learning needs and goals. To facilitate this, the teaching strategy of personal portfolio development may be appropriate. In this approach, rather than students being required to complete specific assignments to achieve a grade in the course, they are asked to develop a personal portfolio to demonstrate their learning in the course. An artist's portfolio contains examples of the artist's work and is used for purposes of promotion. Each of the items in the portfolio has been chosen because it reflects the artist's skill and is representative of his or her style and preferred subject matter.

Similarly, students' portfolios will contain items, or artifacts, that illustrate their individual interests and expertise.

The student-produced artifacts that constitute their portfolios could include scholarly papers, PowerPoint or Prezi presentations, reports, videos, or podcasts. Students individualize their learning within the content scope of the course by deciding what they want to learn and how they are going to show their teacher that they have achieved their personal learning outcomes. Guidelines regarding both the types of assignments required and the level of the assignments (paraprofessional, continuing education, undergraduate, or graduate level) will assist students in creating their portfolios. These guidelines can be framed using questions such as the following: At the end of our course, what would each of you want to have in your portfolio to show others what you can do? What do you most need to know from the field of ____, and how can you create an item, assignment, object, or artifact to illustrate your accomplishments and knowledge?

From the Field: Online Office Hours

Cheryl Crocker uses a variety of communication technologies to be part of the students' networks and to make herself available when they need her. She provides the students with contact information and a designated time each week to reach her through email, texting, instant messaging, Skype, and so on. She initiated this as a way to reduce the number of emails. Office hours are typical in face-to-face teaching, and she thought that they might transpose well to online courses. She holds her official office hours for one hour per week throughout the term and comes online during that specified hour. Students are aware that she is available and meet with her online as they deem necessary. During these meetings, Cheryl guides students in making connections that facilitate their learning and answers questions related to the course and assignments. Student feedback about this approach is primarily positive. Cheryl reports that her office hours are used quite extensively near assignment deadlines and frequently after the return of an assignment.

EMAIL AN AUTHOR

Connectivist thinking encourages learners to reach out to individuals and information sources that are well beyond the confines of their online classroom. A significant requirement of any health care education program is incorporating information from published works to support care decisions. Evidence-informed practice is essential to excellence in health care. While students are probably familiar with publications as information sources, they may not always view the authors of those publications as possible connections as well. Instructors can suggest that students email an author of a publication they found valuable, stipulating that professional communication with an author includes informed comments on the publication, thoughtful questions, and respect for the author's time. If the author's email contact is not included with the publication, students can email the publisher of the book or journal with a request to forward their message to the author.

CONCLUSION

"At its heart," Downes writes, "connectivism is the thesis that knowledge is distributed across a network of connections, and therefore that learning consists of the ability to construct and traverse those networks" (2007, para. 1). Networks are made up of unlimited numbers of nodes that connect to one another in random and ever-changing ways. However, the ways in which these connections occur can form patterns that can be recognized by an individual or a group. Moreover, as Siemens notes, "Networks can combine to form still larger networks (each node in a larger network can be a network of nodes itself). A community, for example, is a rich learning network of individuals who in themselves are … learning networks" (2005, p. 6).

In health care education especially, it is vitally important that learners be able to recognize what they need to know, seek out information from a diverse array of sources, and then organize that information and critically assess its value. Connectivist theory emphasizes these skills and thus helps learners make optimal use of the abundance of information available in a digital world. Connectivist learning is predominantly informal and initiated by students themselves in response to their own interests and needs. This can make measuring student progress and achievement challenging when traditional methods of student assessment are used. Connectivism, with its presumption that a "right" answer today may be wrong tomorrow, offers teachers a fresh point of view for course design, teaching, and student evaluation.

REFERENCES

Barabási, A. L. (2002). *Linked: The new science of networks*. Cambridge, MA: Perseus.

Couros, A. (2009). Open, connected, social: Implications for educational design. *Campus-Wide Information Systems, 26*(3), 232–239.

Downes, S. (2005). An introduction to connective knowledge [blog]. Retrieved from http://www.downes.ca/post/33034

Downes, S. (2006). Learning networks and connective knowledge. Retrieved from http://it.coe.uga.edu/itforum/paper92/paper92.html

Downes, S. (2007). What connectivism is [blog]. Retrieved from http://halfanhour.blogspot.ca/2007/02/what-connectivism-is.html

Gleick, J. (1987). *Chaos: The making of a new science.* New York: Penguin.

Hewitt, J., & Scardamalia, M. (1998). Design principles for distributed knowledge. *Educational Psychology Review, 10*(1), 75–96. doi:10.1023/A:1022810231840

Park, C. L., Crocker, C., Springate, J., Nussey, J., & Hutchings, D. (2010). Evaluation of a teaching tool—wiki—in online graduate education. *Journal of Information Science Education, 21*(3), 313–322.

Pea, R. (1993). Practices of distributed intelligence and designs for education. In G. Salomon (Ed.), *Distributed cognitions: Psychological and educational considerations* (pp. 47–87). New York: Cambridge University Press. Retrieved from http://halshs.archives-ouvertes.fr/docs/00/19/05/71/PDF/A67_Pea_93_DI_CUP.pdf

Rocha, L. M. (1998). Selected self-organization and the semiotics of evolutionary systems. In S. Salthe, G. Van de Vijver, & M. Delpos (Eds.), *Evolutionary systems: The biological and epistemological perspectives on selection and self-organization* (pp. 341–358). Retrieved from http://informatics.indiana.edu/rocha/ises.html

Siemens, G. (2002). Effective teaching [blog]. Retrieved from http://www.elearnspace.org/blog/2002/08/29/effective-teaching/

Siemens, G. (2004). Connectivism: A learning theory for the digital age. Retrieved from http://www.elearnspace.org/Articles/connectivism.htm

Siemens, G. (2005). Connectivism: Learning as network-creation [Word document]. Retrieved from http://www.elearnspace.org/Articles/networks.htm

Siemens, G. (2006). Learning in synch with life: New models, new processes. Google Training Summit. Retrieved from http://www.elearnspace.org/Articles/google_whitepaper.pdf

Siemens, G. (2008). Description of connectivism. Retrieved from http://www.connectivism.ca/about.html

5

Transformational Learning: Creating Attitudinal Shifts in Online Learners

Transformative experiences cause us to think differently and can even alter our cherished assumptions. When our learning is transformative, our perspectives change, our attitudes shift, and we begin to see ourselves and the world around us through new lenses. Learning environments that challenge students to question what they believe to be true and ultimately to interpret information more critically can be transformative. But change is seldom easy for individuals at any stage of their careers. For example, in health care, learners who have not yet served in the field may feel that they have not gained sufficient disciplinary knowledge to question existing assumptions. Learners with experience in health care bring perspectives supported by real-world practice and may come with strongly held beliefs founded on their experiences. Transforming may be difficult for anyone. Kim's story is typical.

Kim is a student in a health disciplines course. She could be a nurse, a social worker, a dietitian, a physiotherapist, an occupational therapist, a chiropractor, a dental hygienist, a radiation therapist, or any other learner involved in providing health care. She could be a novice beginning her program of study or an expert continuing her education in her chosen field.

Kim has always loved school, at every level. She reads professional journal articles of interest and browses the newspaper daily. Since much of what she reads aligns with what she already knows, she seldom has reason to question. Recently, Kim decided to take an online course to, in her words, "keep her thinking." For a course assignment, she was asked to present two perspectives on an issue that was important to her. She had difficulty even thinking of an issue to present. Her upbringing and education taught her to respect the printed word and not to second-guess those who "know." One could describe Kim as content with her existing knowledge and beliefs.

To facilitate Kim moving ahead with the perspectives assignment, her instructor suggested that she consider the issue of "increasing scope of practice in your area of practice." Kim appreciated her instructor's idea, but secretly, she thought, "Who would disagree with that?" She did not see this as a contentious statement: there was only one "right" viewpoint, and it was an obvious one at that.

The first part of the assignment asked Kim to journal her beliefs and attitudes related to her identified issue. Her journal page remained blank. Kim's intentions to complete her assignment remained just that—intentions. What could Kim's online teacher (a practitioner of transformational learning) do to facilitate meaningful shifts in Kim's perspectives?

BACKGROUND THEORY

What Is Transformational Learning?

In the late 1970s, Jack Mizerow began developing a theory of adult learning that he called transformational learning (1978). Transformational learning emerged as a process of critical reflection and rational discourse relating to personal experience. In essence, Mizerow (1981) defines transformational learning as critically reflecting on our assumptions and beliefs and then intentionally creating a new view of the world. O'Sullivan (1999) describes transformative learning as involving a deep shift in consciousness that changes a person's view of his or her place in the world.

Mezirow's theory comprises three dimensions: psychological (changes in how people understand themselves), convictional (changes in belief systems), and behavioural (changes in lifestyle) (Mizerow, 1997). The outcome of transformative learning is what Mizerow (1978) calls "perspective transformation," which he has concluded rarely occurs. When it does occur, perspective transformation is usually triggered by a life crisis and results in a disorienting dilemma for the learner. This traumatic life event triggers the deep conscious reflection that underpins the critical examination that results in transformative learning. In sum, as learners consciously examine underlying views and assumptions of which they may have hitherto been unaware, their view of the world is transformed.

Mezirow claims that some learning experiences have such a strong influence on learners that they can affect all future learning. He writes about "meaning schemes"—beliefs, attitudes, and emotional reactions that are acquired uncritically during childhood. Meaning schemes are "meaning perspectives" that filter future perception and determine the meaning of future experiences (Taylor, 1998).

In much the same way that, in Piaget's theory of child development, the processes of accommodation and assimilation occur naturally, without need for critical thought, Mezirow argues that adult learners are easily able to fit some new experiences into their current meaning perspective or frame of reference. Other experiences, however, particularly personal crises or confusing issues, require reflection and dialogue with others before being incorporated into a transformed meaning perspective.

According to Mezirow (1981), transformational learning is fundamentally a rational and analytical process. In other words, learners change their viewpoint through an active process of critically reflecting on what they believe. Transformational learners need to identify their assumptions, values, and beliefs before they can consciously make a choice to see the world in a new way.

As with any theory, critique of transformational learning is ongoing. Taylor (1997, 2007), for example, questions whether the fundamentals of the model have been fully researched, suggesting that the original model has been applied repeatedly to different situations with limited attention to debate, critique, or building on others' writing. As for whether context has been adequately addressed, Clark and Wilson (1991) assert that Mezirow's emphasis on individual agency has resulted in the neglect of family, peer contexts, and culturally embedded values and mores. Merriam (2004) questions whether all adults can be expected to function at the level of cognitive function needed to reflect critically. She argues that the model is not broadly applicable in that it excludes those with limited ability to think critically and to engage in rational discourse. Some critics question whether perspective transformations actually do include psychological shifts. Tennant (1993), for instance, notes that the shifts or changes in world view described in the theory are based more on cognition than on psychology or emotion.

Responses to these and other critiques are also ongoing. Although Mezirow's original conceptualizations were based on just one small grounded theory study of American women's reflections following their experience of returning to a community college (Marsick & Mezirow, 1978), the theory continues to endure and expand, offering "one of the most generative ideas for both practitioners and researchers" (Dirkx, 2011, p. 139). General publications such as the *Journal of Transformative Education* and *The Handbook of Transformative Learning: Theory, Research and Practice* (Taylor & Cranton, 2012) reflect how the theory is currently being debated, developed, and refined. Discipline-specific publications such as *Transformative Learning in Nursing: A Guide for Nurse Educators* (Morris & Faulk, 2012) reflect applications of the theory in health care education.

As transformational learning theory has continued to evolve, the discussions of educational theorists have been wide ranging, exploring such concepts such as humanism, emancipation, autonomy, equity, self-knowledge, participation, cultural spirituality (narratives developed within students' contexts), positionality, and neurobiology—it has been found that the brain structure actually changes during the learning process (Grabove, 1997; Janik, 2005; Taylor & Cranton, 2012). Discussions addressing the role of emotions, relationships, social contexts, different cultural affiliations, creativity, and the arts continue to impact the evolution of the theory as well (Taylor & Cranton, 2012).

All variations of transformational learning theory emphasize characteristics of instructors and students, course content, learning environments, and instructional activities as important. The contribution of these factors to transformational learning is considered in the following sections. Of note, Taylor (1998) suggests that not all learners are predisposed to engage in transformative learning. The same can be said for teachers, not all of whom may feel comfortable with the goal of transformative learning. In addition, many adult learning situations do not necessarily lend themselves to transformative learning (Imel, 1998).

The Instructor's Role in Transformational Learning

In the transformational learning context, the instructor "functions as a facilitator and provocateur rather than as an authority on subject matter" (Mezirow, 1997, p. 11) and is responsible for creating a learning environment that promotes trust and relationship building. This means encouraging "learners to create norms that accept order, justice, and civility in the classroom and respect and responsibility for helping each other learn; to welcome diversity; to foster peer collaboration; and to provide equal opportunity for participation" (p. 11). Mezirow takes this one step further: "The facilitator works herself out of the job of authority figure to become a colearner" (p. 11). The instructor or facilitator is also responsible for determining the content, or what Anderson, Rourke, Archer, & Garrison (2001) call the "trigger event" that initiates the transformative learning process. Educators attempting to elicit transformational learning create opportunities, both in and outside the classroom, for learners to participate in experiences that bring new insights. Without such experiences to test and explore new perspectives, it is unlikely that learners will fully transform (Taylor, 1998).

The Student's Role in Transformational Learning

Taylor (1998) suggests that Mezirow places too much emphasis on the instructor, thus decreasing the importance of the student's role in critical thinking and discourse leading to transformation. Indeed, as the theory has continued to evolve, theorists such as Kitchenham (2008) and Mezirow himself (2009) have stressed that the transformation comes from the creative and intuitive processes of the student (see also Boyd & Myers, 1988; Grabove, 1997). Boyd and Myers (1988) note that before learner transformation can occur, there may be a need for personality to be changed, consciousness expanded, and ability to discern enhanced; the learner may even have to go through a grieving process. In other words, certain rational and emotional student actions may be essential to transformation (Imel, 1998).

Describing her own transformation as a home economist, McGregor (2004) notes that all transformed learners have their own stories: the transformative experience is a unique journey for each learner. The commonality in the role of the student is an active reflection on foundational assumptions, values, and beliefs. Students need to engage in challenging their conscious and unconscious views and to be open to seeing the world in a different way in order for transformation to be possible.

The Role of the Instructional Environment in Transformational Learning

Three teaching approaches are central to fostering emancipatory transformative learning (Freire & Macedo, 1995), all of which help form the learning environment and determine course content and instructional activities. First, the instructor must make critical reflection central, with the goal of helping learners to rediscover their own power and develop an awareness of agency to transform society and their own realities. Second, a liberating approach to teaching is necessary, an approach couched in "acts of cognition not in the transferral of information" (Freire & Macedo, 1995, p. 67). This is a "problem-posing" and dialogical methodology (p. 70). A third essential approach is that of nurturing a horizontal student-teacher relationship where the teacher works as a political agent and on an equal footing with students (Taylor, 1998, p. 8).

Mezirow (1997) suggests specific instructional techniques and activities to engage students in transformational learning, including journal writing, metaphorical thinking, life history exercises, learning contracts, group projects, case studies, and role playing. Taylor (1998) agrees that reflective journalling, classroom dialogue, and critical questioning are learning activities that have the potential to help students transform.

According to Dirkx (2006), a holistic approach to transformative learning recognizes other ways of knowing (intuition, somatic knowledge) as well as the roles of feelings and relationships with others. Vital to the process of genuine transformation, therefore, are conversations with students about feelings they are experiencing and reasons for their specific decisions in the critical thinking process. The learning environment must be one in which students feel safe engaging in learning activities that require them to reflect on deeply held personal perspectives. If learners are expected to share their perspectives, a supportive learning environment is an essential precursor.

The power imbalance between students and teachers found in some instructional environments may prevent learners from freely expressing themselves. Even if the teacher is attempting to be a co-learner, the inherent power in the position of instructor might intimidate some students, leading them to acquiesce in the teacher's belief system. Hart (1990) notes that Mezirow ignores the power differential in teaching relationships; if transformation is to occur, however, it is crucial to strive for a teacher-learner relationship in which the power differential is as minimal as possible.

Finally, the transformation that results from learner engagement in specific learning activities may be "enduring and irreversible" (Courtenay, Merriam, & Reeves, 1998). The transformation may go beyond an epistemological change in world view; it can also involve an ontological shift (Lange, 2004). True transformational learning can therefore be life changing for students. All parties involved in such a venture need to be aware of the potential upheaval that such learning may have for the students, the teachers, and others affiliated with them. Core views will be challenged and students may feel compelled to make life changes based on their learning. Such potentially transformative endeavours need to be engaged in with eyes open.

TEACHING ACTIVITIES AND STRATEGIES CONGRUENT WITH TRANSFORMATIONAL LEARNING

Transformational learning seeks above all to trigger new insights and to invite critical reflection. Although these goals may sound simple enough, they are not always easy to achieve. The following offers a variety of activities and strategies that educators can use to create attitudinal shifts in online learners.

Triggering New Insights

Transformative learning theorists acknowledge the power of a life crisis or a deeply disorienting dilemma to bring about significant changes in an individual's perspective or way of viewing the world. The insights gained from these shifts in perspective can be life changing. The occurrence of such transformational events is not, however, predictable, and personal crises obviously do not form a routine part of the learning environment. All the same, educators can implement strategies that mimic the sort of fundamental questioning that triggers important new insights. The strategies often centre on requiring students to present topics from different points of view.

FORMAL DEBATE

Because debating requires students either to take on a perspective different from their own or to defend their own views on a topic, a debate can be effective teaching activity for helping students to identify their underlying beliefs, values, and assumptions on a topic, which is an essential beginning step in transformative learning. Adopting a perspective with which one disagrees can trigger a "crisis" and a resulting transformation.

Vandall-Walker, Park, and Munich (2012) give the example of an instructor of a trends-and-issues nursing class who uses debate as a teaching activity that flows through several weeks of the course and includes all students in the course as debaters. In the first week of the course, the students are presented with a list of 25 potential debate topics. In addition, topics not on the original list may be proposed by a group of students. Learners are asked to select from the list three topics that they would like to debate and to prioritize these in order of preference. Students are also given a debate schedule and asked to indicate any particular weeks of the course during which they would not be able fully engage in a debate. Working with the students' choices of topic and the times the students are available, the instructor pairs students and assigns each pair a debate topic. One student in each pair is asked to take the pro side and the other the con side, and the date that the debate will begin is assigned.

Debates are run on a weekly schedule, with one student pair assigned to each week of the course. On the first day of their assigned week, each student in the pair posts his or her side of the debate on a specific discussion forum. Three days later, on the same forum, the two students post their rebuttals to the opponent. The rest of the class is then invited to comment. On the last day of the week, each debater posts a summary statement. Finally, each member of the pair is asked to prepare an individual self-evaluation of his or her performance and experience in the debate and to email the self-evaluation to the instructor.

The debate may be an unsettling experience, even a trigger event, for the students, particularly those who have never participated in a formal debate. Arguing a position in a debate that does not align with one's personal beliefs can provoke anxiety; students are forced to consider perspectives that challenge their own positions.

While instructors do not participate in the debate, they do engage with the students in a general discussion forum about debate and in individual email interactions to attempt to moderate any anxiety before and during the debate process. Debate learning activities are not graded, and no winners or losers are declared. The learning outcomes of the debate are gaining knowledge of course content and learning to express an opinion regardless of whether it is the student's held belief. As part of the debate learning activity, students are introduced to the concept of fallacies of logic and are encouraged to identify fallacies and perhaps to use them when they feel that they do not have strong arguments for their position. At the conclusion of the activity, instructors are encouraged to examine their own perceptions of and views on the use of debates (Park et al., 2011).

As a caution, some might object that obliging students to act in ways that run contrary to their core beliefs—such as expecting them to debate against their own opinions—is unethical. However, the ability to view an issue from more than one side is fundamental to personal and intellectual growth. The transformational learning process may thus require students to enter a state of disequilibrium in which they critically examine their most firmly held values and beliefs. Formalized debate in online courses is one way to achieve this goal.

ONE-MINUTE SELF-DEBATE

For this activity, students are given the following directions for a short solo debate:

1. Listen to the podcast about _____ [a selected course topic], available at _____.

2. Consider the following statement: _____. [The instructor provides a statement related to the podcast that includes at least two obviously different perspectives.]

3. Agree with the statement and write down one point of support for the affirmative position.

4. Disagree with the statement and write down one point of support for the negative position.

5. Rebut your point of support for both the affirmative and negative positions. Repeat this process several times.

6. Share your best point with the class on the online discussion forum created for this purpose.

This shorter version of an online debate learning activity achieves some of the same goals as a formal debate: it helps students to consider both their held viewpoint and alternative perspectives on challenging topics. To achieve this, students need to reflect on what they believe about a topic and consider how others may see this topic differently. Because learners do the one-minute debate privately, they may, through honest reflection and self-examination, uncover deeply held perspectives that they may have been reluctant to share publicly. Additionally, the one-minute debate requires less organizational time on the part of the instructor than the formal online debate described above. The main drawback of the one-minute self-debate is that classmates are not part of the learning activity and shared learning is less likely to occur.

MOOT COURT

Few experiences are as life changing as those that play out in courtrooms. Defence attorneys and prosecutors present arguments that can deeply impact individuals and their families. Impartial judges are expected to weigh evidence that may challenge their own personal beliefs and assumptions. Judges' verdicts must take into account both sides of an argument and apply their knowledge of the law to render a decision.

The courtroom process can be transferred to a "moot court" activity focusing on a relevant health care issue such as assisted suicide.

Online students are randomly assigned to the role of defence attorney, prosecutor, and judge. This way, students may find themselves in the position of preparing a life-saving defence for an individual accused of an action that they find abhorrent—a situation that could trigger a transformative process. Defence attorneys and prosecutors must prepare their cases, and the judges their verdicts, within an instructor-specified time limit. Students share their cases and verdicts online in written or video format. Teachers may wish to build in opportunities for debriefing, since personal memories related to the justice system could resurface as students engage in the activity.

PAIR-SHARE: TWO PEOPLE, FOUR VIEWS

For this activity, students are invited to read a scholarly article on a course topic and then to email another student to organize a pair-share discussion on this topic. Students can use online conferencing, e-meeting resources, instant messaging, Skype, or another avenue of communication for their pair-share collaboration. Students reflect on their own perspective on the article, contemplate alternative views on the topic, and then share with their partner at least two viewpoints related to the topic. Instructors can encourage students to practice active listening when their partner is sharing. At the conclusion of the pair-share discussion, the students reflect on their own perspectives and those of their partner and journal about what they discovered.

Inviting Critical Reflection

Before a shift in attitude can be expected to occur, learners must critically reflect on assumptions they believe are true. Because challenging these assumptions, at both a cognitive and an emotional level, can be difficult, the process is unlikely to be spontaneous. Instead, instructors must provide learners with opportunities to question their views on specific ideas or issues. Activities in which no "right" or "wrong" interpretations exist can stimulate critical reflection.

METAPHORICAL THINKING

Since metaphors can encourage critical reflection, introducing students to a metaphor related to a course topic can expand their perspectives and contribute to transformational learning. For example, on the topic of mentoring, the metaphor of a garden as an effective mentoring relationship could be used. If the class is related to leadership, a leader might be seen as the ringleader in a circus. After the metaphor is introduced, students are asked to draw on what they have learned about the topic in the class to write a short comment that extends the metaphor. Each comment begins with a phrase provided by the instructor, such as "An effective mentor-mentee relationship is like a garden because . . ." or "An effective leader is like the ringleader in a three-ring circus because . . ." The student comments are then shared with the class in a discussion forum created for this purpose. A general class discussion evolves from the postings of the comments on the metaphor. The seemingly simple metaphor exercise encourages students to reflect more deeply on a given topic and how it may relate to them.

WHICH PATIENTS WOULD I CHOOSE?

Deeply held values, whether we are aware of them or not, are our blueprints for action. Activities that cause students to examine their values are essential to transformational learning. This exercise can facilitate a values examination.

To begin, the instructor devises a one-page list of approximately 20 patients who have fictitious names and short bios and who require care in the field in which the learners are (or will be) employed. For example, if the class comprises a group of undergraduate student nurses, the list could include bios like the following:

Bill Barker   A 57-year-old gruff-talking man who has been admitted for prostate enlargement and follow-up examinations. Bill often swears and has been noted to speak roughly to his wife, who visits regularly.

Jane Ogdon   A 48-year-old woman who has completed treatment for breast cancer and has been admitted for reconstruction surgery. Her partner, Mary, visits regularly.

Elsie Paul   A 89-year-old woman who has dementia and has been admitted because she has fallen often at home. Her children are not able to help with her care, so she is awaiting placement in long-term care.

Sam Slip   A 28-year-old man who lives on the streets and has been admitted for liver problems and treatment of malnutrition.

Cammy Jones   A quiet and withdrawn teenager who has been admitted because of extreme weight loss and suspected anorexia and bulimia.

Students are given the list of bios and asked to select the five patients they would choose as health care professionals if they had the option to choose. Of course, as health care professionals, we usually do not have this choice, but for the transformative purposes of this exercise, students are asked to make choices. They are also asked to identify five patients they would choose *not* to care for if they had a choice. They then consider why they made the choices they did and record any common themes in their choices. After working on their choices individually, students form small groups and share their observations about their choices as well as what they learned about their once "hidden" values and biases.

This learning activity works effectively online since students receive the bio list in digital form and can engage in either a real-time discussion via e-meeting software or an asynchronous discussion forum. Students find that this learning activity reveals conscious and unconscious beliefs and values that may influence the care they provide. Recognizing these values and beliefs can be an initial step in transformational learning.

From the Field: "The Paths I've Walked"

Sharon Moore created an arts-based pedagogical activity called "The Paths I've Walked," a slide show with images, primarily of nature, set to a tranquil piece of music. Software such as Moviemaker can be used to create such a presentation. In Sharon's case, the intent of this practice is to help students understand the characteristics and tenets of qualitative research. She was inspired to create the slide show while writing a graduate course on advanced qualitative methods. During her preparations, she read an article by McAllister and Rowe (2003), who write, "Being a qualitative researcher involves attributes such as compassion, passion, integrity, tolerance of ambiguity, willingness to play with ideas, knowledge and inquiry, commitment to viewing the social world from the viewpoints of the people being studied, valuing of detail, and willingness to inject something of themselves into the research process and its outcomes" (p. 296). The authors suggest implementing creative teaching approaches using narrative, poetry, dance, film, music, and photographs.

Sharon's four-minute presentation is included via a link near the beginning of the online course. Students are asked to view the presentation, respond in a discussion forum to some related questions that Sharon has incorporated into the presentation, and make some observations about qualitative research based on their classmates' responses.

Sharon has received many positive responses from students about the presentation, which has had some unintended side-effects. The presentation usually comes at a time in the semester when the workload is heavy and the students are feeling stressed. One student remarked, "Thank you Sharon for sharing this slide show with us! I found the images and the music to be very calming and inspirational." Another student wrote, "It forced me to stop and appreciate the world around me in the midst of a hectic schedule."

But the slide show also accomplishes Sharon's primary purpose. One learner remarked, "We each bring to our interpretations of this slide show our own experiences and beliefs. There is not a right or wrong interpretation. All of our contributions are important. The richness in this information is that it considers the perceptions of all of us. Together all this information gives the qualitative researcher a rich and robust collection of information." Still another learner made this observation: "I viewed the slide show late at work one night when I thought the office was empty and accordingly turned the sound quite high. Within minutes a few nurses and clerical staff were drawn from hither and thither by the haunting Celtic melody. As we watched the slide show together I was struck by how one image affected so many people differently or how one image elicited a similar response. It occurred to me that everything we do in qualitative research in contextually based."

CONCLUSION

Transformational learning is about shifts in attitude. Health care students all bring deeply seated and well-established beliefs and assumptions to their learning. Facilitating genuine change in students' views of the world is not easy. Teachers must provide content and experiences that have the potential to trigger new insights and invite critical reflection. Jack Mezirow, a key contributor to the development of transformational learning theory, emphasizes the importance of providing challenges within the educational process. Teachers who challenge learners provide them with opportunities to question commonly accepted truths and to reflect critically on points of view that are different from their own.

Ultimately, however, it is learners themselves who must be open to new perspectives. Although the process of shifting attitudes can be exciting, it can also be disorienting. Students must be active and willing participants throughout the process of transformation.

REFERENCES

Boyd, R. D., & Myers, J. G. (1988). Transformative education. *International Journal of Lifelong Education, 7*(4), 261–284.

Clark, C., & Wilson, A. (1991). Context and rationality in Mezirow's theory of transformative learning. *Adult Education Quarterly, 41*(2), 75–91.

Courtenay, B., Merriam, S. B., & Reeves, P. M. (1998). The centrality of meaning-making in transformational learning: How HIV-positive adults make sense of their lives. *Adult Education Quarterly, 48*, 65–84.

Dirkx, J. M. (2006). Engaging emotions in adult learning: A Jungian perspective on emotion and transformative learning. In E. W. Taylor (Ed.), *Teaching for change: New directions for adult and continuing education* (pp. 15–26). San Francisco: Jossey-Bass.

Dirkx, J. M. (2011). An enduring and expanding legacy. *Journal of Transformative Education, 9*(3), 139–142.

Freire, P., & Macedo, D. P. (1995). A dialogue: Culture, language, and race. *Harvard Educational Review, 65*(3), 377–402.

Grabove, V. (1997). The many facets of transformative learning theory and practice. In P. Cranton (Ed.), *Transformative learning in action: Insights from practice* (pp. 89–96). *New Directions for Adult and Continuing Education, 74.* San Francisco: Jossey-Bass.

Hart, M. (1990). Critical theory and beyond: Future perspectives on emancipatory education. *Adult Education Quarterly, 40*(3), 125–138.

Imel, S. (1998). *Transformative learning in adulthood.* Columbus, OH: ERIC Clearinghouse on Adult Career and Vocational Education, ERIC Digest No. 200. Retrieved from http://calpro-online.org/ERIC/docs/dig200.pdf

Janik, D. S. (2005). *Unlock the genius within: Neurobiological trauma, teaching, and transformative learning.* Lanham, MD: Rowman and Littlefield Education.

Kitchenham, A. (2008). The evolution of John Mezirow's transformative learning theory. *Journal of Transformative Education, 6*(2), 104–123.

Lange, E. (2004). Transformative and restorative learning: A vital dialectic for sustainable societies. *Adult Education Quarterly, 54*, 121–139.

Marsick, V., & Mezirow, J. (1978). *Education for perspective transformation: Women's re-entry programs in community colleges.* New York: Center for Adult Education, Teachers College, Columbia University.

McAllister, M., & Rowe, J. (2003). Blackbirds singing in the dead of night? Advancing the craft of teaching qualitative research. *Journal of Nursing Education, 42*(7), 296–303.

McGregor, S. (2004). Transformative learning: We teach who we are. *Kappa Omicron Nu Forum, 14*(2). Retrieved from http://www.kon.org/archives/forum/14-2/forum14-2_article4.html

Merriam, S. B. (2004). The role of cognitive development in Mezirow's transformational learning theory. *Adult Education Quarterly, 55*(1), 60–68.

Mezirow, J. (1978). Perspective transformation. *Adult Education Quarterly, 28*(2), 100–109. doi:10.1177/074171367802800202

Mezirow, J. (1981). A critical theory of adult learning and education. *Adult Education Quarterly, 32,* 3–23.

Mezirow, J. (1997). Transformative learning: Theory to practice. *New Directions for Adult and Continuing Education, 74,* 5–12.

Mezirow, J. (2009). An overview on transformative learning. In K. Illeris (Ed.), *Contemporary theories of learning: Learning theorists in their own words* (pp. 90–105). London and New York: Routledge.

Morris, A. & Faulk, D. (2012). *Transformative learning in nursing: A guide for nurse educators.* New York: Springer.

O'Sullivan, E. (1999). *Transformative learning: Educational vision for the twenty-first century.* Toronto: University of Toronto Press. Retrieved from http://wiki.sugarlabs.org/images/8/8a/O%27Sullivan19xxch8.pdf

Park, C. L., Kier, C., & Jugdev, K. (2011). Debate as a teaching strategy in online education: A case study. *Canadian Journal of Learning and Technology, 37,* 3.

Taylor, E. W. (1997). Building upon the theoretical debate: A critical review of the empirical studies of Mezirow's transformative learning theory. *Adult Education Quarterly, 48*(1), 34–59.

Taylor, E. W. (1998). *The theory and practice of transformative learning: A critical review.* Information Series no. 374. Columbus, OH: ERIC Clearinghouse on Adult, Career, and Vocational Education.

Taylor, E. W. (2007). An update of transformative learning theory: A critical review of the empirical research (1999–2005). *International Journal of Lifelong Education, 26*(2), 173–191.

Taylor, E. W., & Cranton, P. (Eds.). (2012). *The handbook of transformative learning: Theory, research and practice*. San Francisco: Jossey-Bass.

Tennant, M. (1993). Perspective transformation and adult development. *Adult Education Quarterly, 44*(1), 34–42.

Vandall-Walker, V., Park, C. L., & Munich, K. (2012). Outcomes of formal online debating in graduate nursing education. *International Journal of Nursing Education Scholarship, 9*(1), 1–14. doi:10.1515/1548-923X.2450

6

Quantum Learning Environments: Making the Virtual Seem Real in the Online Classroom

Katherine Janzen

Online classrooms are composed of teachers and students interacting within a virtual medium. This virtual "classroom" can seem like an artificial environment to students—one where reality simply does not exist. At least for some students, the experience of online learning amounts to sitting in front of a computer screen in solitude. In this classroom of one, individual students may never experience a sense of belonging to a larger community. Reduced to feeling invisible, unable to make the much-needed face-to-face connections with one another and with their instructors, students can easily feel isolated and disengaged from the learning experience. As instructors, how can we make students' online experiences seem more real and ultimately more pedagogically effective?

The quantum perspective on learning has recently emerged in the educational literature as a means of bridging the virtual and the real (Janzen, Perry & Edwards, 2011b). In what follows, I will explain how the assumptions and principles of quantum learning, along with supporting literature, can help online teachers to develop "living" environments within the online educational milieu. In addition, I will examine the way in which artistic pedagogical technologies (Perry & Edwards, 2010), as well as other online teaching practices, can be used to promote a sense of reality in the virtual classroom.

BACKGROUND THEORY

Simply put, quantum learning (QL) suggests that the process of learning mimics the behaviour of electrons. QL is based on the idea that, like electrons, everything that exists is connected, or entangled, and is superposed on itself (Bohm 1971, 1973). For example, a giant sheet of cotton fabric exists as a whole despite the individual properties of the cotton threads that bind the fabric together. When looking at the fabric, we are normally not cognizant of each individual thread; rather, we see it holistically, as indivisible. What we see are the patterns in the fabric: the colours, the shapes, the texture—those things that make the fabric real to us. If we saw the fabric merely as individual threads, we may doubt the reality of the existence of the fabric as a whole. The fabric would not be real to us. Likewise, students looking at the virtual environment may only see the individual threads. If they do not find ways to discover or connect the threads in their learning environment, they may never experience a feeling of reality and belonging.

If all that exists is conceptualized as a giant fabric where everything—from quarks to the cosmos—is part of that fabric (connected and entangled) and is constantly communicating no matter where the parts are positioned within that fabric (superposition), then learning is part of that time-space continuum. Students, instructors, and educational institutions become key players within that fabric, which interfaces with the learning environment (Janzen, Perry & Edwards, 2011a). Thus, in QL, learning and learning environments are determined to be holistic in nature, existing as holographic environments.

Assumptions and Principles of Quantum Learning

QL is based on five assumptions and seven principles. The assumptions are:

1. Learning is multidimensional.

2. Learning occurs in various planes simultaneously.

3. Learning consists of potentialities that exist infinitely.

4. Learning is both holistic and holographic and is patterned within holographic realities.

5. Learning environments are living systems. (Janzen et al., 2011a, p. 64)

The principles are:

1. Online learning needs to be multidimensionally constructed. If it is accepted that humans are holistic beings, then learning must be able to reach the learners' multiple dimensions.

2. Online learning must occur in various planes or dimensions in order to access holistic development. Reaching the learner simply in one quantum dimension (e.g., cognitive or social) is not sufficient to promote

learning that extends beyond the confines of the online classroom. Learning that reaches multiple dimensions becomes learning that is accessed for life.

3. Humans have infinite potential to learn and develop in all dimensions.

4. Human potential for learning is ubiquitous. Geographic separation and asynchronous learning are not limits in online learning.

5. Online instructional design should encourage learners to reach beyond temporality and virtuality into holographic realities. Holographic realities, which encourage interaction between and among learners, instructors, the learning environment, and technology, become the essence of holistic online education.

6. Online learning environments are living systems that grow, evolve, and develop through the passage of time and space. Online learning environments are dynamic spaces that support the needs of learners, instructors, and educational institutions.

7. Online learning can result in transformation for teachers, learners, and the educational environment. Ultimately, through this transformation, technology is potentially both directly and indirectly transformed. (Janzen et al., 2011a, pp. 64–65)

The principles of QL can give educators and course designers direction in making the virtual seem real for students in the online classroom.

QL suggests that the virtual and the temporal are inextricably connected. These connections exist ubiquitously and form a primary construct in the educative environment (Janzen et al., 2011a). As learners discover connections that exist between entities, virtual environments become more real. Going back to the metaphor of the fabric, as students are able to conceptualize these discovered connections, the fabric (or their experience as part of the totality of their existence) becomes strengthened and indivisible. Learner experiences become real in their interactions with each other and with the course content. Ultimately, it is through teaching strategies that connect the virtual and real-world environments that reality is infused into online learning environments.

These virtual learning environments, or quantum learning environments (QLEs), become living systems that grow, adapt, and evolve (Janzen et al., 2011a). All that exists within QLEs—students, instructors, and course content—can also grow, adapt, and evolve as online courses progress (Janzen, Perry, & Edwards, 2011c). In QLEs, as in life, growth is a part of the system. This sense of growth or change is one aspect that contributes to making the learning environment real. Artistic pedagogical technologies (Perry & Edwards, 2010) are examples of teaching strategies that help to develop QLEs in online courses.

Artistic Pedagogical Technologies

Artistic pedagogical technologies (APTs) are arts-based online teaching practices that utilize elements of the literary, visual, musical, or dramatic arts. APTs differ from traditional teaching techniques, such as the lecture, because of the emphasis on aesthetics and creativity. Since the concept of APTs was first described, several studies have demonstrated that these teaching strategies benefit online learning (Beth Perry, 2006; Perry, Dalton & Edwards, 2009; Perry, Menzies, Janzen & Edwards, 2011). More specifically, APTs contribute to the development of online learning communities by initiating, motivating, sustaining, and enhancing interactions among students and between students and instructors (Perry & Edwards, 2010). APTs and

QLEs are connected in that the use of APTs in the online classroom contributes to making online classrooms real. Janzen et al. (2011b) found that in classrooms where the APT of photovoice (PV) was used, PV supported students, engaged their interest, and helped to make their interactions more authentic. By examining aspects of APTs and discussing those aspects in light of the virtual learning environment, additional understandings regarding how virtual environments can become real are possible.

Humans are multidimensional. Persons explore their individual and collective worlds sensually, intellectually, socially, culturally, and spiritually. Over the last few decades, this exploration has increasingly included technology. For most people, technology has permeated all aspects of their lives including learning. The Web and social networking sites stand as a testament of this. To the digital native, technology is real. In the online environment, optimal learning embraces multidimensionality.

One of the goals of online learning and QL (as well as APTs) is to reach the students' multiple dimensions. APTs help facilitate learning that can be relevant and meaningful to a wide variety of students and to instructors. In many ways, APTs create living environments that grow in depth and breadth as online courses progress. These learning environments are not flat, one-dimensional environments; rather, they exist as holograms.

Holographic learning environments, or QLEs, facilitate each student's unique and personally meaningful connection to the broader educative world. We are usually most comfortable and most free to be ourselves in our homes surrounded by people who love us. The same comfort level, which promotes effective learning, can be created when students experience the personalization that arises from QLEs.

APTs help create QLEs. Elements of APT learning activities are often familiar to students. For example, they may include photographs of familiar images, poems, literature, and/or musical selections that are personally meaningful to individual students (Perry &

Edwards, 2010). Seeing the familiar embedded in the unfamiliar (new knowledge in an online course) helps make learners feel more comfortable in their personalized learning environment. Such a state supports meaningful learning.

In some ways, the arts-based nature of APT teaching activities touches the humanity of students and calls out to them first as human beings and then as learners. Art is a human creation and is infused with human emotion. Through the connections that students make to course content while participating in APT activities, personal memories are elicited, which may in turn engender new understandings. The APTs and subsequent learning can then be integrated into students' lives. The learning environment and the learning become more tangible.

APTs help create positive, safe learning environments in which students can explore and share emotions appropriately. Janzen et al. (2011b) found that during APT activities, emotion was evoked and frequently shared. The sharing of emotion creates context for students as they navigate through online courses. The comfort and familiarity created by APTs, combined with the emotions they evoke, help members of the learning community (including the instructor) to see one another as real beings with hopes, fears, and dreams. This recognition acts as a springboard to connecting the personal with the educative.

APTs take the familiar and apply it to the educative realm, which may not be so familiar and which can be a bit frightening at times. Most people are apprehensive when beginning an educative endeavour. For example, looking at a course outline can evoke fear as students comprehend all that they will have to do in a few short weeks of instruction. APTs lessen apprehension by inviting the students to be "at home." This can help create an invitational educational environment (Purkey & Novak, 2007) that makes learning more possible.

Thinking of this in another sense, hospitalized children often have a toy or a blanket from home that calms them and connects them to home. Likewise, the elderly in a hospital setting may cling to a familiar object that brings them comfort. While hospitalization can be a scary experience, the stuffed animal or item from home becomes the conduit to a less traumatic experience. Similarly, APTs are a conduit to safety and a sense of comfort in the online educative classroom. APTs, given their familiarity, may create online environments where students feel they are at home in some sense. Gradually, the concept of "home" can be magnified in the learning environment as students interact with the instructor and other students and, in doing so, genuinely become known to one another. APTs can be the catalysts for these interactions.

Consider the idea of hanging pictures on a wall. People hang pictures because they feel a connection with them; they have meaning and purpose in our lives. APTs are like hanging pictures up on the walls of our minds. The pictures provide frames of reference. Similarly, APTs are, in many ways, like grade school "show and tell," but these learning activities require deeper levels of critical thinking and analysis. The "show and tell" is yet another connecting experience. The responses of students to APTs are really explications of their own worlds and how their worlds connect with what they are learning. Carter and Click (2006) note that when virtual environments "mimic real life, [students] become more enmeshed with the content" (p. 2). Enmeshing with content could be likened to connecting.

The concept of play is important in QL. APTs encourage students to play. Children learn naturally through play. As people grow older, most lose that capacity to play, since life stressors often suppress playfulness. There is little time left over to play. APTs invite learners to play as a route to learning in part because play is another way of being at home within the educative milieu and playing provides a connection between the personal and the educative. In APTs, students are invited to play with the activity, play with the thoughts and feelings that the activity evokes, and, ultimately, engage in arts-based play with the other students. Playing together for the purpose of forming connections and learning helps create a sense of community in online courses. This feeling of community is considered important to positive learning outcomes in online learning (Carter & Click, 2006).

TEACHING ACTIVITIES AND STRATEGIES CONGRUENT WITH QUANTUM LEARNING

This section describes selected APTs, along with other teaching techniques that can be easily used in the online classroom. These strategies can effectively contribute to making the virtual seem more real for students. Each activity draws upon a familiar construct and uses that construct in new ways that are conducive to online learning and to creating QLEs.

"Haiku It"

Many students were taught the technique of writing Japanese haiku poetry in elementary school (University of Missouri, 2009). The "Haiku It" APT (Perry, Janzen, & Edwards, 2011) asks students to summarize a course concept in a haiku in order to make the concept personally meaningful. The concept can be taken from an individual unit of the course, or it can be an overarching concept drawn from the entire course. A haiku consists of three lines, the first line having five syllables, the second line having seven syllables and the remaining line having five syllables. The lines of the poem do not rhyme.

"Haiku It" encourages students to be concise as they create their own haikus. In order to be concise, students need to have a very clear understanding of the key elements related to a given concept. Additional benefits of writing haiku are developing academic literacy and finding one's inner voice (Iida, 2011). The following is an example of a haiku written by a student in an online course about research dissemination strategies. The poem summarizes the key ideas that the student considered important at the conclusion of the course and demonstrates that the learner had grasped essential understandings related to the course learning outcomes:

> We share our voices.
> Our words extending farther
> As the world listens.

It may be helpful at the beginning of a haiku activity for the instructor to model the activity by providing examples. Haikus written by students from a previous offering of the course or composed by the instructor may give students confidence in writing their own haikus while also providing a refresher on the format of a haiku. Because this APT may not appeal to all students, some of whom may have an aversion to writing poetry, this activity should be optional. However, even those who do not write a haiku may benefit from reading poems created by their classmates.

While some might argue that writing poetry is not appropriate in a course other than English literature, it should be noted that haiku writing is transferable to all subjects. There is precedence in the academic world regarding the value of haikus as an academic exercise. Specifically, searching the term "dissertation haiku" reveals an amazing collection of haikus created by scholars who have summarized their PhD dissertations in haikus.

Conceptual Quilting

The activity of quilting has been found to have individual as well as group benefits. Burt and Atkinson (2011) conducted a series of interviews with members of a Glasgow quilting group and summarized their results as follows:

> Cognitive, emotional and social processes were uncovered, which participants identified as important for their wellbeing. Participants found quilting to be a productive use of time and an accessible means of engaging in free creativity. Colour was psychologically uplifting. Quilting was challenging, demanded concentration and participants maintained and learned new skills. Participants experienced "flow" while quilting. A strong social network fostered the formation of strong friendships. Affirmation from others boosted self-esteem and increased motivation for skill development. (p. 1)

Conceptual quilting in the virtual classroom may embody some of the same benefits as physical quilting (Beth Perry, 2006).

The APT of conceptual quilting is an online activity that can be done individually or with the entire class. All students are familiar with quilts that are constructed using a collection of individual "squares" or pieces. As an individual activity, conceptual quilting involves students creating an online virtual quilt with the e-squares in the quilt representing important concepts that students have learned or take-home messages they have heard. Students can use software such as Microsoft Word or PowerPoint to construct their quilts. The quilts are then shared with the instructor and other students on a forum set up for that purpose. Students can "walk through" this virtual quilt gallery and view their classmates' quilts. This activity is an excellent summary learning activity for students since it causes them to reflect on what they have learned. Additionally, in viewing the quilts prepared by others, they may remember concepts other than those included in their own quilts.

A variation on conceptual quilting is collaborative quilting. When done as a collective activity, the class is divided into groups and each group member contributes a quilt square toward that group's finished virtual quilt, which is then presented on an online forum. A short explanation of the quilt accompanies the virtual quilt.

This activity promotes socialization and group cohesion, much like physical quilting does. The finished collaborative quilt is a representation of the diverse viewpoints of those in the class community. Themes may emerge from the various quilt pieces provided, and the class as a whole may engage in a thematic analysis on a discussion forum as part of the collective quilting activity.

A second variation on conceptual quilting is the word quilt. Some learners may lack the necessary technical skills to use graphics and online images to create quilts. The option of creating a word quilt could be offered to these learners. Students compose their word quilt in a word-processing document and can add creativity by using different fonts and sizes. Although the word quilt requires less technical skill on the part of the learner, similar learning outcomes can be achieved.

Progressive Poetry

Humans having expressed themselves using poetry for millennia, and it is an important genre in the Hebrew scriptures (Bliss Perry, 2008). Hebrew poetry, like the APT of progressive poetry (Perry et al., 2011), uses a "structure ... where one idea and phrase is balanced against another" (Bliss Perry, 2008, p. 92). In the online classroom, the APT of progressive poetry consists of the instructor either choosing an existing poem or writing a poem on a course theme or topic. This poem is then posted to an online forum. Students respond to the instructor's poem by writing a poem themselves, adding another stanza to the opening poem, or sharing a poem that they have found. Regardless of which option they choose, their addition must expand on the ideas presented in the initial poem in some way. The teacher may than add a response to the student's contribution by adding another poetic phrase or stanza to the collaborative piece. Complex topics and ideas become more fully understood as the authors add to the initial stimulus poem.

As an example, the first poem given below is the instructor's poem posting, "The Road Not Taken," by Robert Frost, originally published in 1916 and now in the public domain. An example of a possible student contribution to the progressive poem follows. In order to respond to the instructor's poem, the student must comprehend the key message in the poem, link course learning to this understanding, engage in personal reflection related to these ideas, and compose a succinct and relevant poetic contribution. These may all be course learning outcomes.

Poem Posted by the Instructor

The Road Not Taken

Two roads diverged in a yellow wood,
And sorry I could not travel both
And be one traveler, long I stood
And looked down one as far as I could
To where it bent in the undergrowth;

Then took the other, as just as fair,
And having perhaps the better claim,
Because it was grassy and wanted wear;
Though as for that the passing there
Had worn them really about the same,

And both that morning equally lay
In leaves no step had trodden black.

Oh, I kept the first for another day!
Yet knowing how way leads on to way,
I doubted if I should ever come back.

I shall be telling this with a sigh
Somewhere ages and ages hence:
Two roads diverged in a wood, and I—
I took the one less traveled by,
And that has made all the difference.

<u>Student Poem</u>

The Roads I Travel

In my life I have travelled many roads.
Some well-trodden
Where others sing the praises of sights seen
And the view of the many becomes
Jumbled into communal experience.

On these roads
I conquer the required.

But I have travelled other roads
Barely visible to those who pass by.
These are the quiet paths
Where agony and ecstasy
Are my companions.

Within these paths
I conquer myself.

Morning Coffee Forum

The ritual of drinking morning coffee is one of life's simple pleasures. Sharing a cup of coffee with others not only gets us started in the morning but also provides "innumerable moments of good conversation and congeniality" (Ayers, 1995, February, para. 3). The morning coffee learning activity can be undertaken in several ways within an online course for a variety of educational purposes. For example, to open a course and encourage conversation and socialization, students may be invited to join a "morning coffee" introductory forum. On this forum, they post a brief profile describing themselves and their interests and explaining why they are taking that particular course. Class members are invited to comment on their classmates' postings.

As a variation, the morning coffee forum can be used in online group work. Once the student groupings are determined, each group initially meets for "morning coffee," where the members engage each other with their ideas and get to know one another on a more personal level than may be possible on the main online forum. This "morning coffee" meeting can take place on a closed private forum created specifically for the group, or students can meet for coffee using social meeting software such as Skype.

In another variation of this activity, students are invited to make the morning coffee experience more tangible by sharing a photo of their favourite coffee cup (with a sentence or two about "their" cup) as part of the e-coffee experience. In sharing these images, students often reveal details about themselves in a very natural way that facilitates students getting to know one another. For example, one student posted a photo of her Canadian Blood Services mug. In a conversation with another student in her group , she shared that she supported this organization because her child had a blood disease and required blood products. Another student's coffee cup was made of English bone china, which gave her the opportunity to talk about her English heritage. All of these personal details might be easily disclosed in a face-to-face coffee meeting but are hidden in the virtual world unless images of personal coffee cups are shared.

Course Climate Checks

The climate is not only a topic of everyday conversation; it also tends to guide our lives to a great extent. If we live in a cold climate, we layer clothing appropriately. Those in rainy climates grab an umbrella before heading outdoors. Likewise, online courses have learning climates that develop over time and are subject to change, depending on the needs of individuals or groups of students. Affirmative course climates have been found to "have a positive effect on student satisfaction" and to influence learning in a positive way (Belfer, 2000, p. 1265).

A course climate check provides an opportunity for students to offer feedback to their instructors about the climate of the course. The student responses in this activity help instructors to create and maintain a positive learning environment, which may, in turn, aid learners in achieving course outcomes.

In a course climate check, each student is invited to write a paragraph relating a climate-related metaphor to their personal experience of the course. The instructor begins the activity by suggesting an initial statement like, "The course is like being in a hurricane because . . ." or "The course is warm and sunny because . . ." Students finish the sentence and provide an additional explanation of the initial statement. Student responses are shared privately with the instructor.

As a variation, students may come up with their own initial statement and expand on it in the paragraph. The activity can be conducted at strategic points during the course such as at the beginning, during particularly stressful points, or at the end. The activity provides instructors with the opportunity to determine which students might be struggling with the course and allows them the chance to take preemptive action to assist particular learners. If the tone of most or all of the student responses is negative, this can prompt the instructor to modify his or her approach to try to improve the learning climate and the student learning experience.

In another variation, students are provided with a graphic of a thermometer and asked to give a temperature value related to how they are experiencing the course. Are they "cold," signifying that they are unmotivated and uninspired? Are they "hot," indicating that they are overwhelmed and stressed by the course activities and assignments? Or do the students report that they are "just right," suggesting that the course has engaging learning activities, a favourable class climate, and effective instruction?

"Begin with Baroque"

Baroque music from composers such as Bach, Pachelbel, Vivaldi, and Handel has been found to stimulate the production of alpha waves in the brain, which has positive effects on human memorizing and learning (Gao, Ren, Chang, Liu, & Aickelin, 2010). Baroque music has 50 to 70 beats per minute, which mimics the human heart rate (Highland Council, 2006). When used in the educative environment, baroque music has been found to lower blood pressure, increase encoding and memory, amplify spatial awareness, potentiate concentration, enable inspiration, and further reading and language abilities (Amerson, 2006; Gao et al., 2010).

Instructors can use "Begin with Baroque" in several ways in the online environment. Students can be invited to play a selection of baroque music (via a link provided by the instructor) while engaging in required readings or assignments, or, in courses that require reflective journalling (Amerson, 2006), while writing in their journal. One of the many websites that students can access for free baroque music is "A Baroque Banquet" at http://www.baroquecds.com/baroquebanquet.html, which offers many selections by various composers.

Gratitude Letters

The expression of gratitude has many benefits. Emmons (2010), a world leader in gratitude research, found that in addition to experiencing physical and psychological benefits, individuals who express or cultivate gratitude in their lives reap social benefits, including the reduction of feelings of being isolated. This finding has applicability in the online classroom, where students may feel educationally isolated due to geographic separation and the often asynchronous nature of online learning. Since "gratitude may in fact be a positive, universal characteristic that transcends historical and cultural periods" (Emmons & Shelton, 2002, p. 460), gratitude may also influence real-world and virtual environments positively, making students' experiences and relationships with other members of the class more real and less distant.

In the gratitude letters activity, students are invited to compose gratitude letters to classmates of their own choosing. The gratitude letters could express appreciation for what another student taught them, comments on a particularly inspirational posting, or a remark on how learning with the chosen classmate benefited the writer personally and/or academically. The writer then emails the gratitude letters to the selected recipients. Gratitude letters work well as a closing activity in online classes. Instructors could also compose gratitude letters to each of the students expressing affirmation and an appreciation for the contributions of each student during the course. The instructor can personalize each letter by referring to individual students' specific contributions to the course, thus making the communiqués more meaningful. Instructor involvement in this learning activity ensures that all students receive at least one gratitude letter.

As a variation of the gratitude letters activity, students can be encouraged to share letters of gratitude with people outside the course: authors of journal articles or books that they have found useful in the course or friends, family members, or mentors who helped them succeed during the course.

Virtual Talking Sticks

Within the traditions of some Aboriginal communities of North America, the talking stick is a sacred symbol and provides an opportunity for members of a community to share their voices and wisdom (Thunderbird, n.d.). When one member of the "talking circle" holds the talking stick and speaks, all others engage in "active listening." Using the talking stick reflects the participants' respect for "harmony, balance and good manners among humans, the Great Mystery and Mother Earth. The Talking Stick is a symbol of respect for the thoughts, stories and individual histories of each member participating in the circle." Individuals speak "their truth in a place of confidence and safety." The stick is then passed to the next person, who, if he or she chooses to speak, has uninterrupted time to do so. All members of the talking circle have the opportunity to both speak and listen, and both of those actions are equally valued.

In online learning environments, virtual talking sticks provide opportunities for students to share their truths and perspectives in an uninterrupted way. The purpose of a virtual talking stick on an online forum is twofold. First, students have the opportunity to actively reflect as they prepare and share what they wish to "talk" about on the virtual talking stick forum; second, other students learn to listen actively and absorb what is virtually spoken without having to think about preparing a response, since the talking circle is not "a debating society" or a place for dialogue (Thunderbird, n.d.). As each student "speaks," the individual knows that what is shared will be received with respect and confidentiality.

Virtual talking sticks can be used in several ways within online courses. As described above, a "virtual talking stick" forum can be created where students are invited to create threads about what they are discovering on a certain course topic. When one student is finished "speaking," he or she would virtually hand over the talking stick by naming the next "speaker," who would then post on the forum. Since students never know when the stick might be handed to them, they might be motivated to log in to the discussion forum often to see whether the stick has been handed their way. This process of talking and handing over would continue until all students have had the opportunity to "speak." In a variation on this activity, students can share YouTube videos and podcasts rather than, or in addition to, a piece of writing.

Another way of using the virtual talking stick is for the instructor to take the lead in presenting thoughts about a certain topic. To start this process, the instructor posts an image of a talking stick with a short description of its history, meaning, and use. The instructor then chooses a topic and posts his or her own thoughts and impressions, which constitute the first "speaking." Then the instructor passes the talking stick to a named student. This modelling of the process gives class members an idea of how the virtual talking stick forum is to proceed. The named student either chooses to share his or her perspective on the designated topic or passes the stick to another chosen student. This process of speaking (or choosing not to speak) and passing the stick to another student proceeds until everyone in the class has had a chance to speak in the forum.

The virtual talking stick forum could be particularly effective in a final course offering before graduation. In this instance, students are invited to share how they envision their future as graduation nears. The virtual talking stick provides an opportunity for both self-assessment and deep reflection. This type of forum could ultimately become a gift for students as they venture into the world of their chosen profession.

Classroom Eulogy

Eulogies create spaces where individuals meet for one last time. Sir Andrew Motion, former poet laureate of the United Kingdom, describes a eulogy as "at once a greeting and a letting go" (Motion, 2013, p. 4). For students and instructors, the ending of an online course can involve a grieving process as students say goodbye to fellow students and instructors. Due to geographical separation and the asynchronous nature of online courses, the paths of class members may never cross again after a course ends. If a sense of community has formed during the online course, class participants may experience a sense of loss at the end of the course, and deliberate closing activities may be useful. Furthermore, through such closing activities, students may be motivated to reflect on what they learned, which may help to consolidate learning.

Classroom eulogies create spaces where students can reflect on the course content and on the relationships they have formed. They allow students an opportunity to review and consolidate their online experiences, making them more real to themselves and to fellow students. By giving students one final chance to reflect, individually and collectively, on the course content and on the online relationships that have developed, a classroom eulogy may decrease the anxiety that comes with transitions and endings.

Classroom eulogies can take many forms. Students can post a photo of a piece of art that they have created, a photographic image, a poem, a motto, a favourite saying, a short story, a piece of music, or a quotation that summarizes their experiences and learning in a course, along with a paragraph explaining their choice.

Alternatively, students can follow an instructor-provided template for a classroom eulogy. Themes for such a template might include the following:

- Thinking big: the highlights of the course

- Thinking small: the little things that were most meaningful

- Thinking sad: the challenges and/or difficulties that arose during the course

- Thinking happy: moments of pleasure or accomplishment

- Thinking inside: what students will take away from the course, the key relationships that were formed and why these relationships were valuable

- Thinking outside: how the future may unfold (Cooperative Group Ltd., 2013, p. 6)

CONCLUSION

At times, online students are left feeling that their online experience is simply not "real." Online learners can feel very alone and isolated from classmates and instructors. Interactions with the computer screen may become the sum of their online learning experience. To reduce this possibility, online instructors can use teaching techniques and activities that are designed to engage students and to help reduce this sense of remoteness. These approaches are founded on what is familiar to students; that familiarity is applied to course activities.

The quantum perspective on learning provides a theoretical foundation to support the need for developing quantum learning environments. Artistic pedagogical technologies, which are based on the five principles of quantum learning, can help to create such environments. The benefits of using APTs include providing the opportunity to play, presenting an opportunity for authentic communication, making multiple connections between the real-world and the virtual, finding a personal and collective voice, feeling at home in the online milieu, and ultimately empowering students, who feel valued, respected, and needed as they contribute to the course. The culmination of this chapter is found within the nine teaching activities presented. These activities offer instructors ways to make their online classrooms come alive—helping the virtual environment to become a "living," dynamic learning space. Reality is infused into virtual environments by using familiar activities, constructs, or concepts that most students have experienced in their everyday lives. Through the recognition and use of these familiar activities, which have been adapted to the online classroom, students (health care professionals and others) may come to experience a virtual learning experience that feels like "home" and is a comfortable, welcoming space for each of them to grow, explore, and learn.

REFERENCES

Amerson, R. (2006). Energizing the nursing lecture: Application of the theory of multiple intelligence learning. *Nursing Education Perspectives*, 27(4), 194–196.

Ayers, E. (1995, February). The history of a cup of coffee. *San Diego Earth Times*. Reprinted from *World Watch*, September/October 1994. Retrieved from http://www.sdearthtimes.com/et0295/et0295s1.html

Belfer, K. (2000). A learner centred assessment of quality for online education: Course climate. In J. Bourdeau & R. Heller (Eds.)., *Proceedings of World Conference on Educational Multimedia, Hypermedia and Telecommunications 2000* (pp. 1265–1267). Chesapeake, VA: AACE. Retrieved from http://www.editlib.org/p/16251

Bohm, D. (1971). Quantum theory as an indication of a new order in physics. Part A: The development of new orders as shown through the history of physics. *Foundations of Physics, 1*(4), 359–384. doi:10.1007/BF00708585

Bohm, D. (1973). Quantum theory as an indication of a new order in physics. Part B: Implicate and explicate order in physical law. *Foundations of Physics, 3*(2), 139–168. doi:10.1007/BF00708436

Burt, E. L., & Atkinson, J. (2011, June 5). The relationship between quilting and wellbeing. *Journal of Public Health.* Retrieved from http://jpubhealth. oxfordjournals.org/content/early/2011/06/05/pubmed.fdr041.abstract

Carter, B., & Click, A. (2006). Imagine the real in the virtual: Experience your second life. *Proceedings of the 22nd Conference on Teaching and Distance Learning,* 1–4. Retrieved from http://www.uwex.edu/disted/conference/ resource_library/proceedings/06_4202.pdf

Emmons, R. A. (2010). Why gratitude is good. Retrieved from http://greatergood. berkeley.edu/article/item/why_gratitude_is_good/

Emmons, R. A., & Shelton, C. A. (2002). Gratitude and the science of positive psychology. In C. R. Snyder and S. J. Lopez (Eds.), *Handbook of positive psychology* (pp. 459–471). New York: Oxford University Press.

Gao, H., Ren, Z., Chang, X., Liu, X., & Aickelin, U. (2010). The effect of baroque music on the PassPoints graphical password. *Proceedings of 2010 ACM Conference on Image and Video Retrieval,* 129–134.

Highland Council. (2006). *Learning to learn.* Retrieved from http://www. highland.gov.uk/learninghere/supportforschoolstaff/ltt/issuepapers/ learningtolearn.htm

Iida, A. (2011). *Revisiting haiku: The contribution of composing haiku to L2 academic literacy development* (Doctoral dissertation, Indiana University of Pennsylvania). Retrieved from http://dspace.iup.edu/bitstream/ handle/2069/359/Atsushi%20Iida.pdf?sequence=3

Janzen, K. J., Perry, B., & Edwards, M. (2011a). Aligning the quantum perspective of learning to instructional design: Exploring the seven definitive questions. *International Review of Research in Open and Distance Learning, 12*(7), 56–73. Retrieved from http://www.irrodl.org/index.php/irrodl

Janzen, K. J., Perry, B., & Edwards, M. (2011b). Becoming real: Using the artistic pedagogical technology of photovoice as a medium to becoming real to one another in the online educative environment. *International Journal of Nursing Education Scholarship*, 8(1), 1–17. doi:10.2202/1548-923X.2168

Janzen, K. J., Perry, B., & Edwards, M. (2011c). A classroom of one is a community of learners: Paradox, artistic pedagogical technologies, and the invitational classroom. *Journal of Invitational Theory and Practice*, 17, 28–36.

Motion, Andrew. (2013). Foreword to *Well chosen words: How to write a eulogy*. Retrieved from http://www.co-operative.coop/Funeralcare/brochures/march2013/Well-chosen-words/files/inc/bdca2b53b8.pdf

Perry, B. [Beth]. (2006). Using photographic images as an interactive online teaching strategy. *The Internet and Higher Education*, 9(3), 229–240. doi:10.1016/j.iheduc.2006.06.008

Perry, B., Dalton, J., & Edwards, M. (2009). Photographic images as an interactive online teaching technology: Creating online communities. *International Journal of Teaching and Learning in Higher Education*, 20(2), 106–115. Retrieved from http://www.isetl.org/ijtlhe/pdf/IJTLHE302.pdf

Perry, B., & Edwards, M. (2010). Creating a culture of community in the online classroom using artistic pedagogical technologies. In G. Veletsianos (Ed.), *Emerging technologies in distance education* (pp. 129–151). Edmonton: Athabasca University Press.

Perry, B., Janzen, K. J., & Edwards, M. (2011). Creating invitational online learning environments using art-based learning interventions. *eLearning Papers*, 27, 1–4. Retrieved from http://www.elearningeuropa.info/en/node/111106

Perry, B., Menzies, C., Janzen, K. J., & Edwards, M. (2011). The effect of the artistic pedagogical technology called photovoice on interaction in the online post-secondary classroom: The teachers' perspective. *Ubiquitous Learning: An International Journal*, 2(3), 117–128.

Perry, B. [Bliss]. (2006). *A study of poetry*. Charleston, SC: BiblioBazaar (Original work published 1920).

Purkey, W. W., & Novak, J. M. (2007). *Inviting school success: A self-concept approach to teaching, learning, and democratic practice*. Belmont, CA: Wadsworth.

Thunderbird, S. (n.d.). *Sacred symbols and their meanings.* Retrieved from http://www.shannonthunderbird.com/Native_contributions.htm

University of Missouri. (2009). Writing poetry for elementary grade levels. Retrieved from http://ethemes.missouri.edu/themes/1398

Conclusion:
Rethinking Online Course Design and Teaching

This book provides an overview of contemporary and emerging educational theories that have the potential to underpin course design and online teaching. In addition to reviewing the central elements of each theory, specific teaching strategies congruent with each theory are described. Our goal is that educators of health professionals, both novice and expert, will review the theoretical perspectives and consider using the presented teaching practices in their online teaching. Furthermore, we anticipate that by understanding the theories that give rise to the teaching techniques and activities presented, readers will know why and when specific practices work and will create new activities that will help students to achieve their learning outcomes.

We believe that to be effective, online courses and teaching have to be different from traditional face-to-face education. For example, teaching online requires deliberate actions and strategies to help course participants feel like members of an actual (real) class community. In traditional classrooms, the grounds for establishing a sense of community occur naturally because of geographic proximity. In cyberspace, this natural association is not necessarily present, and teachers need to take steps to make themselves real to students and to help students become real to one another. We have presented many teaching practices that can be used to achieve this outcome.

Here, we bring together broad "lessons learned" in making online courses more engaging. Fundamentally, we acknowledge that online courses can have an abundance of wonderful teaching strategies and activities and yet can still be a failure. The teacher matters. Online teachers face unique challenges. How can an online teacher with a toolkit of excellent teaching techniques ensure success? How can teachers in the online medium transcend the emptiness of cyberspace to become real to students? How can educators create learning environments where classmates become as tangible to one another as if they were sitting side by side in a face-to-face classroom? We address some of these questions by providing online teachers with important take-away messages.

LESSON I: START WITH THEORY

The temptation is to start with the product. In online teaching, the desired product for some teachers could be an innovative, creative learning activity that students will be motivated to participate in and rate as transformative. But the first step in designing successful learning activities is to consider how and why activities are effective. Teachers need to consider what they believe about teaching and learning; in other words, they need to know which educational theory aligns with their perspective and preferred teaching processes. This alignment is important in structuring learning activities that are congruent with their teaching style and course design. A misalignment in teaching approaches and learning activities may confuse learners and result in a learning environment where students are unsure of teacher expect-ations. If students receive mixed messages (for example, the teacher invites them to propose their own assignments and then imposes set assignments on them), they may become uncertain, their motivation may decrease, and they may lose focus on their course work. Teachers who know which educational theory underpins their course design and instruction and then follow through with approaches that align with it provide learners with a sense of security that ultimately enhan-ces learning and teaching.

LESSON 2: TAKE RISKS

What we have learned in our years of teaching online, echoed by the colleagues who provided "From the Field" teaching experiences, is that truly exemplary online teaching is a high-risk activity, at least in the beginning. Individuals are naturally reluctant to change, and teachers are no different. For centuries, education has been primarily lecture based with the teacher knowing more than the students and imparting this knowledge to receptive vessels. However, the online learning milieu and the technology that supports it offer many new avenues to acquire and share knowledge. Furthermore, since the nature of the learner has changed, we must rethink how education and teaching are perceived. Knowledge is within all of us and access-ible by everyone. The teacher is no longer seen as the "all-knowing" person but rather as a co-creator of knowledge and a guide who helps learners to assess available knowledge to determine the relative cred-ibility of information.

With this role change, the traditional approach to teaching is no longer as effective. Whether instructing paraprofessionals or postdoc-toral scholars, today's online health care teachers need to take risks and try new ways of teaching to align with the learning needs of stu-dents. This risk-taking means shedding the protective security of the top-down lecture format where teachers are held in high esteem and not questioned. Effective online teachers need to be open to learning and becoming active participants in dynamic online learning environments.

LESSON 3: CRAFT A PLAN

Good planning is the foundation of success for most things in life, and achieving excellence as a teacher is no different. After reading this book, you are equipped with an abundance of teaching ideas grounded in educational theory. If the book works as we hope it does, you will be inspired to identify and learn about the educational theory that underpins your teaching values and practices. We invite you to review the suggested teaching strategies and imagine how you could use many of these (or variations of them) in your own teaching. But there is one more step—you need to create a plan. A teaching plan, while important to success, is really quite simple: it follows the common steps of assessment, planning, implementation, and evaluation.

Begin your plan with assessment. Ask questions such as, Who are your learners? Where are they in their program of study? What do they already know? Why were they motivated to choose this particular career in health care? And how are they most likely to be able to demonstrate what they know? Assess your curriculum and professional knowledge in relation to the resources and freedoms that you have. For example, at first glance, some online curricula may seem to have little room for introducing additional teaching techniques. Yet despite this apparent limitation, we invite you to consider some of the activities and approaches that we have suggested and to personalize required curricula by introducing those that fit for you. Assess the nature of your learning milieu. Think about the experiences and events that are occurring in your program and in students' personal

Conclusion

lives. Imagine how linking these experiences to online activities might help make your virtual classroom feel more real. Perhaps most importantly of all, assess your strengths and limitations as a teacher. In planning, consider which educational theory is consistent with your teaching philosophy and goals, and the learning outcomes you hope to achieve. Select a variety of teaching techniques and activities that will help students achieve required learning outcomes and grow as professionals. Be sure to think beyond the approaches that naturally seem to fit within your own world view. For example, teachers who feel particularly comfortable with an invitational theory approach might intentionally plan to stretch their repertoire by including transformational learning activities in their teaching plan. In planning to use a particular online teaching activity, be sure to consider questions such as, How much time will I need to utilize it? Where will it fit best in the course? What resources do students need to employ it? And how will it enhance students' ability to assimilate needed and relevant professional knowledge?

As you implement the techniques you have chosen, remember that the best plans all require some modification as the unanticipated happens. Be open to needed changes and accept that some teaching approaches in some situations simply may not work as expected. Throughout the process of implementing any activity, make a point of continually reflecting on your teaching practice. In his seminal book *The Reflective Practitioner*, Donald Schön (1983) coined the term "reflection in action" as a way of explaining how professionals develop their expertise. As Schön suggests, throughout your teaching practice, reflect on the teaching strategies you've chosen and used, and make frequent refinements to your plan.

Finally—remember to evaluate your unique teaching plan. Curricula will require you to evaluate your students' progress, and most courses in health care programs include class evaluation forms. In addition to these formal evaluation opportunities, question both yourself and your students about what went well and what elements of your teaching practice could be improved. What surprised you? What kinds of unexpected learning occurred in your online class? How might insights gleaned from this incidental learning be incorporated into future teaching plans?

LESSON 4: STUDENTS AND TEACHERS ARE PEOPLE

Even though in the online learning milieu, teachers and students can literally be learning together while on different continents, never having exchanged eye contact or a handshake, online teachers and learners are still people. People are much more than two-dimensional photographs or online avatars. People have emotions, fears, insecurities, desires, and suspicions. People are people. These elements of being human should not be ignored in developing effective online courses or in online teaching. To ignore these human qualities in students is to destine online teaching to failure, or at least to being lacklustre. Rather, effective online teachers recognize the humanness in each learner and individualize their teaching to embrace and build on these realities.

Furthermore, teachers are people too. To be effective, teachers need to develop self-awareness of their own idiosyncrasies that impact their teaching. These unique qualities make teachers distinctive, and those with insight into themselves are able to both communicate these to learners (helping to establish their authenticity with students) and build on what they know about themselves as they develop and employ their teaching skills.

LESSON 5: WE ARE IN THIS TOGETHER

Teaching has changed: teachers are now learners, and in many ways, learners are teachers. The vast mount of ever-changing knowledge on a subject now available with a few keystrokes means that no one person can ever know everything on a topic. Even if one person has an extensive knowledge base, that knowledge is continually challenged and expanded by incessant research happening in real time. Our first point is that teachers need to be open to being unceasing learners, willing to revise what they "know" and add new emerging knowledge to their mindset.

Our second point is that learners are often very well versed in their subject areas. They have instant access to many sources of information on their specific topic. In online learning communities, students often teach classmates and teachers what they know about a topic. Online education is taking place in a more democratic environment where all participants have an equal role in sharing, assessing, re-forming, deconstructing, and creating knowledge.

In our work with students and teachers from a variety of different health disciplines, we have come to trust the process of learning that occurs when students and teachers come together. Whether in brick-and-mortar buildings or virtual classes, our students come with the expectation that activities have been designed to further their professional knowledge. The stakes are high and students are heavily invested in achieving the skills, knowledge, and attitudes necessary to practice in their chosen profession. They are both informed and dedicated. When teachers bring subject-matter expertise, passion for their field, and an enthusiastic belief that learning will happen, students and teachers can genuinely feel they are "in it together."

Conclusion

LESSON 6: TEACHING MATTERS

Whether you are teaching online, in a blended course, or face to face, teaching matters. In *The Courage to Teach*, Palmer (2007) writes that "good teachers share one trait: a strong sense of personal identity infuses their work" (p. 11). He goes on to explain:

> Good teachers possess a capacity for connectedness. They are able to weave a complex web of connections among themselves, their subjects, and their students so that students can learn to weave a world for themselves. The methods used by these weavers vary widely: lectures, Socratic dialogues, laboratory experiments, collaborative problem solving, creative chaos. The connections made by teachers are held not in their method but in their hearts—meaning *heart* in its strictest sense, as the place where intellect and emotion and spirit and will converge in the human self. (2007, p. 11)

In short, *"good teaching cannot be reduced to technique; good teaching comes from the identity and integrity of the teacher"* (2007, p. 10; italics in original). Although teaching has changed with the advent of online education, a good teacher still makes a difference to learners and to the learning process itself. The difference is visible in learning outcomes, particularly in the degree of excitement and engagement that students experience while taking the class, and is partly the result of the familiar qualities of a good teacher—the ability to explain ideas clearly, for example, or to pose thought-provoking questions, or to offer criticism in a constructive and encouraging manner. To a degree, however, what makes a good teacher is something more elusive and nebulous. It is a way of being that cannot be readily quantified or even adequately conveyed in words: it can be experienced, but it resists articulation.

Conclusion

Think about your own teachers who you recall as exemplary. What was it about these people that made their teaching outstanding? It was probably not the inventiveness of their learning activities or their firm foundation in educational theory but rather who they were as human beings and how they related to you as a student. We can write books, do research, make conference presentations, and try to teach people to teach. We are convinced that everyone can become a better educator. But there is something more—something that Palmer has captured, at least in part. As he puts it, "in every class I teach, my ability to connect with my students, and to connect them with the subject, depends less on the methods I use than on the degree to which I know and trust my self—and am willing to make it available and vulnerable in the service of learning" (2007, pp. 10–11).

We challenge online educators and course designers to consider taking deliberate actions to enhance the effectiveness of their online courses. We challenge you to learn about educational theory, to take risks and try some of the learning activities in this book and even invent some of your own. Furthermore, we challenge you to consider Parker's words and examine how your intellect, emotion, and spirit come together to make you the teacher you are and the teacher you will become.

REFERENCES

Palmer, P. (2007). *The courage to teach: Exploring the inner landscape of a teacher's life* (10th anniversary ed.). San Francisco: John Wiley.

Schön, D. (1983). *The reflective practitioner: How professionals think in action.* New York: Basic Books.